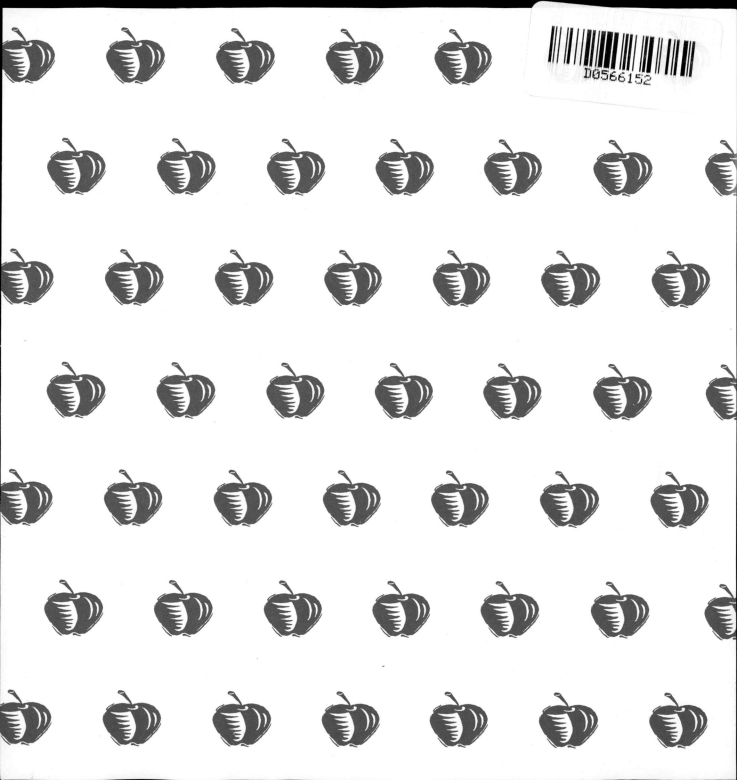

Better Homes and Gardens®

Healthy Meals
fast

Pictured on the cover: Pasta Primavera with Salmon (see recipe, *page 43)*

Healthy Meals *Fast*

Project Editor: Lois White
Project Designer: Nancy Wiles
Contributing Copy Editor: Winifred Moranville
Test Kitchen Director: Sharon Stilwell
Production Manager: Ivan McDonald

Vice President, Publishing Director: John Loughlin
Publisher: Mike Peterson
Editor-in-Chief: Don Johnson
Design Director: Jann Williams

All of us at Meredith Corporation are dedicated to providing you with the information and ideas you need to create tasty foods. We welcome your comments and suggestions. Write to us at: *Healthy Meals Fast,* Meredith Custom Publishing, 1912 Grand Ave., Des Moines, IA 50309-3379.

Nutritional Facts
To help you keep track of what you eat, each recipe in this book lists nutritional values for one serving. Here's how we made our analyses: When a recipe gives a choice of ingredients (such as chicken or turkey), we use the first choice in our analysis. Ingredients listed as optional were omitted from our calculations. Finally, all values were rounded to the nearest whole number.

CONTENTS

No matter how busy you are, there's no need to sacrifice great-tasting weeknight meals that are healthful, too. Whether you have 15, 20, or 30 minutes, one of our good-for-you main dishes is sure to meet the demands of your schedule and your diet. And, best of all, each recipe takes advantage of healthful, convenient products and common seasonings that are easy to find in the supermarket.

To begin, check the nutrition facts with the recipes—you'll find the recipes are moderate in calories, fat, cholesterol, and sodium so they fit into a healthy diet. Then, sample a few recipes. We think you'll agree: Healthful eating doesn't get any easier—or more delicious—than this!

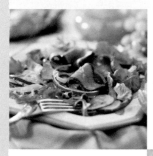

15-Minute Meals
Page 4

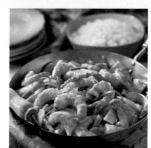

20-Minute Meals
Page 26

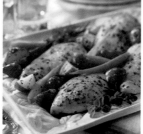

30-Minute Meals
Page 60

Special-Day Meals Page 84

Recipe Index Page 95

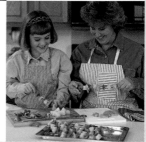

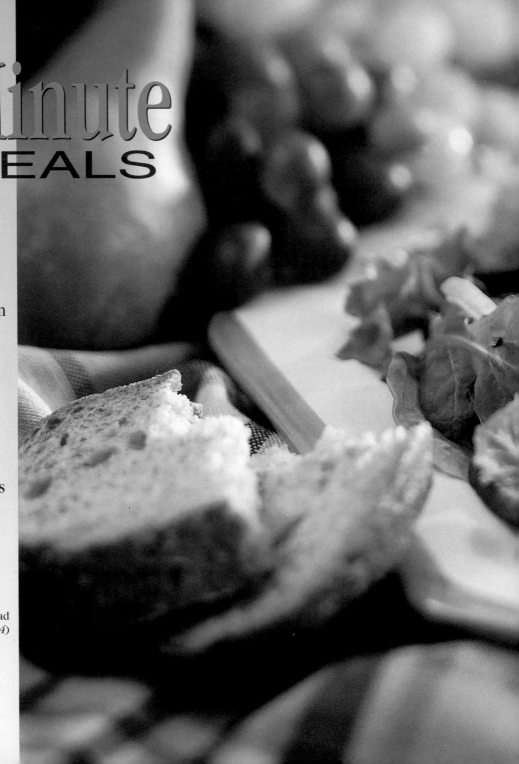

15-Minute MEALS

No time to cook? There's an easier, healthier, and more satisfying solution than your neighborhood fast-food restaurant. In these recipes, good nutrition and great taste go together in 15 minutes. That's less time than it would take to get to a restaurant and back!

Garden Beef Salad
(see recipe, *page 24*)

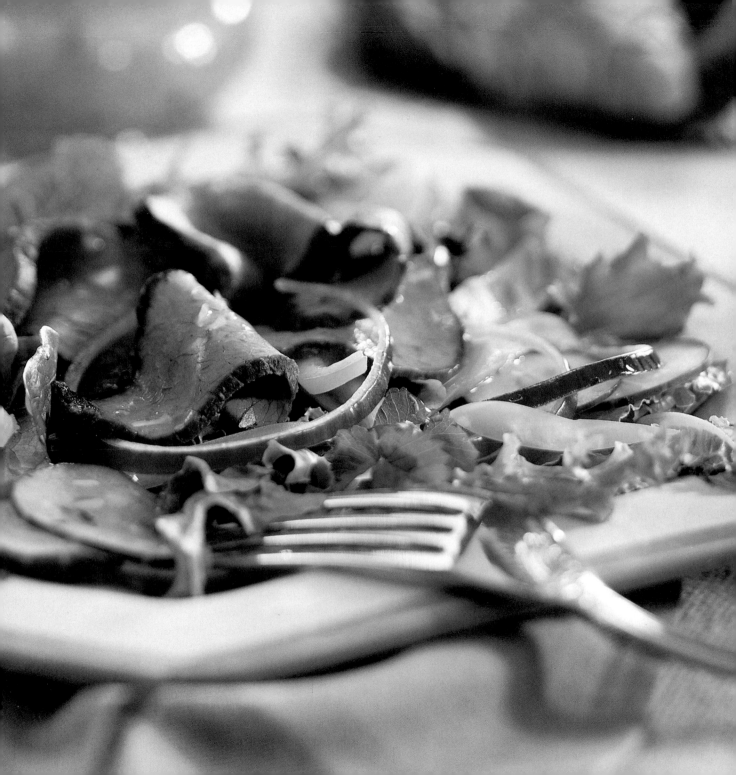

TEX-MEX CHICKEN TOSTADAS

4	7-inch flour tortillas
	Nonstick spray coating
12	ounces ground raw chicken
2	teaspoons chili powder
1	8-ounce can reduced-sodium tomato sauce
2	tablespoons salsa
2	medium tomatoes
1⅓	cups shredded lettuce
⅓	cup shredded reduced-fat cheddar cheese

◆ **Place** tortillas in a single layer on a baking sheet. Spray with nonstick coating. Place in a cold oven. Set oven to 450°. Bake for 10 to 12 minutes or until crisp and lightly browned.

◆ **Meanwhile,** cook and stir chicken and chili powder in a large skillet over medium heat until chicken is no longer pink. Stir in tomato sauce and salsa; heat through. Chop the tomatoes. Spoon the chicken mixture onto tortillas. Top with lettuce, tomatoes, and cheese. Makes 4 servings.

NUTRITION FACTS PER SERVING: 282 calories, 20 g protein, 29 g carbohydrate, 9 g fat, 48 mg cholesterol, 2 g dietary fiber, 347 mg sodium.

HERBED CHICKEN SANDWICHES

4	small skinless, boneless chicken breast halves (12 ounces total)
	Nonstick spray coating
½	cup fat-free cream cheese
½	teaspoon dried dillweed
⅛	teaspoon garlic powder
4	hamburger buns, split, *or* 8 slices whole grain bread
¼	of a medium cucumber

◆ **Rinse** chicken; pat dry. Place chicken between 2 sheets of plastic wrap; pound with the flat side of a meat mallet to flatten slightly. Sprinkle chicken with ¼ teaspoon *pepper.* Spray an unheated 12-inch skillet with nonstick coating. Preheat over medium heat. Add chicken; cook for 8 to 10 minutes or until tender and no longer pink; turn once.

◆ **Meanwhile,** stir together cream cheese, dillweed, and garlic powder in a small bowl. Spread cut sides of buns with cheese mixture. Thinly slice cucumber. Place cucumber slices on bun bottoms. Top with chicken. Add bun tops. Makes 4 servings.

NUTRITION FACTS PER SERVING: 357 calories, 27 g protein, 45 g carbohydrate, 7 g fat, 49 mg cholesterol, 2 g dietary fiber, 445 mg sodium.

ZESTY FRIED CHICKEN

    2 tablespoons cornmeal
    1 teaspoon paprika
    ½ teaspoon salt
    ½ teaspoon garlic powder
    ½ teaspoon pepper
    ¼ teaspoon ground cumin
    4 medium skinless, boneless chicken breast halves (1 pound total)
       Nonstick spray coating

◆ **Combine** cornmeal, paprika, salt, garlic powder, pepper, and cumin in a shallow dish or on a sheet of waxed paper.

◆ **Rinse** chicken (do not pat dry); coat chicken evenly on all sides with the cornmeal mixture.

◆ **Spray** an unheated large skillet with nonstick coating. Preheat skillet over medium heat. Add chicken; cook for 8 to 10 minutes or until tender and no longer pink, turning occasionally to brown evenly on all sides. Makes 4 servings.

NUTRITION FACTS PER SERVING: 141 calories, 22 g protein, 4 g carbohydrate, 4 g fat, 59 mg cholesterol, 0 g dietary fiber, 321 mg sodium.

EATING RIGHT: A BALANCING ACT

There are no "good" foods or "bad" foods in a sound diet. Eating right is a matter of balance. Here's how you can tip that balance in your favor.

• Eat a variety of foods.

• Eat at least 5 servings of fruits and vegetables per day.

• Eat just 5 to 7 ounces of lean meat, poultry, or fish per day.

• Choose foods low in fat, saturated fat, and cholesterol.

• Use lower-fat dairy products, such as skim milk and lower-fat cheeses.

• Enjoy high-fat, high-calorie foods in moderation.

• Include more fiber-rich foods—such as whole grain products, fruits, vegetables, and dried beans—in your diet.

• Use sugar and salt in moderation.

• Drink the equivalent of 8 to 10 cups of water per day.

• Limit the amount of alcohol you consume.

• Balance your caloric intake with regular, moderate exercise.

GLAZED CHICKEN AND GRAPES

    4   medium skinless, boneless chicken breast halves (1 pound total)
        Nonstick spray coating
    ¾   cup seedless red *or* green grapes
    3   fresh parsley sprigs
    ⅓   cup apple jelly
    2   tablespoons dry sherry *or* dry white wine
    2   teaspoons lemon juice

◆ **Rinse** chicken; pat dry with paper towels. Spray an unheated large skillet with nonstick coating. Preheat the skillet over medium heat. Add chicken breasts; cook for 8 to 10 minutes or until tender and no longer pink, turning once. Transfer chicken to serving plates. Cover to keep warm.

◆ **Meanwhile,** cut the grapes in half and snip the parsley. Add the apple jelly, dry sherry, lemon juice, ¼ teaspoon *salt,* and dash *pepper* to the skillet. Cook and stir just until the jelly is melted. Add the halved grapes and snipped parsley. Heat through. Spoon jelly mixture over chicken. Makes 4 servings.

NUTRITION FACTS PER SERVING: 221 calories, 22 g protein, 24 g carbohydrate, 4 g fat, 59 mg cholesterol, 0 g dietary fiber, 193 mg sodium.

HOISIN BROILED CHICKEN WITH CASHEWS

    1   cup quick-cooking rice
    ½   cup loose-pack frozen peas
    4   medium skinless, boneless chicken breast halves *or* turkey breast
        tenderloin steaks (1 pound total)
    2   tablespoons hoisin sauce
    2   tablespoons dry roasted unsalted cashew halves and pieces
    2   green onions, sliced (¼ cup)

◆ **Set oven** to broil. Prepare rice according to package directions, *except* omit salt and margarine; stir peas in with rice.

◆ **Meanwhile,** rinse chicken; pat dry. Place chicken, boned side up, on the unheated rack of a broiler pan. Stir together hoisin sauce and 2 teaspoons *water* in a small bowl. Brush chicken with hoisin sauce mixture. Broil 4 to 5 inches from the heat for 7 minutes. Turn; brush with sauce. Broil 5 to 8 minutes more or until chicken is tender and no longer pink. Serve over rice mixture. Top with nuts and onions. Makes 4 servings.

NUTRITION FACTS PER SERVING: 271 calories, 25 g protein, 28 g carbohydrate, 5 g fat, 59 mg cholesterol, 1 g dietary fiber, 227 mg sodium.

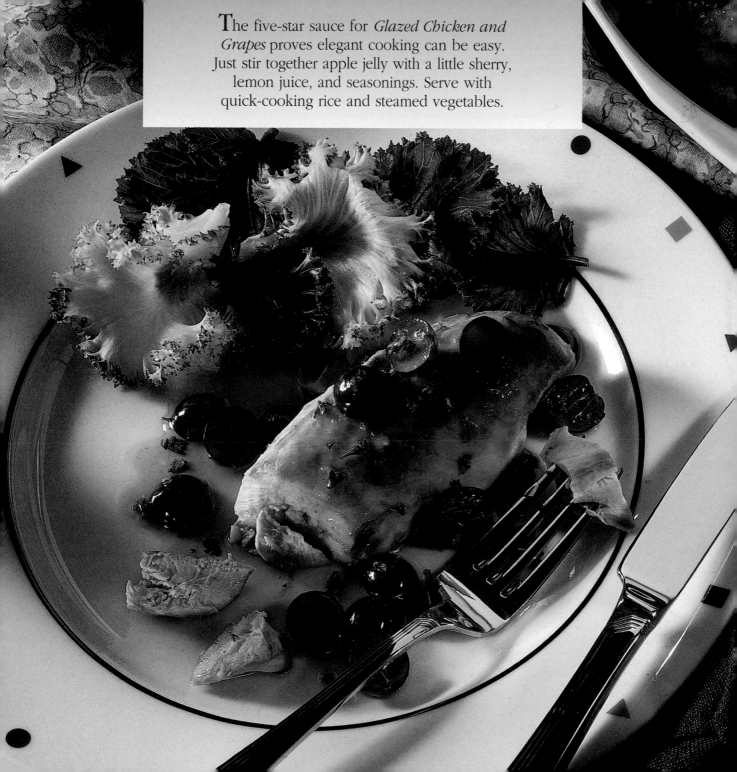

The five-star sauce for *Glazed Chicken and Grapes* proves elegant cooking can be easy. Just stir together apple jelly with a little sherry, lemon juice, and seasonings. Serve with quick-cooking rice and steamed vegetables.

BALSAMIC CHICKEN WITH ZUCCHINI

Balsamic vinegar, aged several years in a wooden barrel, lends its full-bodied flavor to this super-simple skillet dinner.

¼ cup fat-free Italian salad dressing
1 tablespoon balsamic *or* red wine vinegar
1 teaspoon sugar
4 medium skinless, boneless chicken breast halves (1 pound total)
  Nonstick spray coating
2 medium zucchini, bias sliced ¼-inch-thick
2 teaspoons cooking oil
4 Roma tomatoes, quartered

◆ **Stir** together salad dressing, vinegar, and sugar in a small bowl; set aside. Rinse chicken; pat dry with paper towels. Slice each chicken breast half lengthwise to make 4 strips.

◆ **Spray** an unheated 12-inch skillet with nonstick coating. Preheat skillet over medium heat. Add zucchini; cook and stir for 3 to 4 minutes or until zucchini is crisp-tender. Transfer to a serving platter. Cover to keep warm.

◆ **Heat** oil in the same skillet over medium-high heat. Add chicken; cook and stir for 3 to 4 minutes or until chicken is tender and no longer pink. Transfer chicken to serving platter.

◆ **Stir** tomatoes and dressing mixture into skillet. Cook and stir about 30 seconds or until heated through. Spoon over chicken and zucchini. Makes 4 servings.

NUTRITION FACTS PER SERVING: 164 calories, 22 g protein, 7 g carbohydrate, 5 g fat, 59 mg cholesterol, 1 g dietary fiber, 271 mg sodium.

SAFFRON CHICKEN AND RICE

Start with a cooked rice-and-vegetable combination from your deli down the street, season it with saffron, and you'll get a paella-like flavor from across the world.

  3 cups purchased cooked rice with vegetables
  ½ to ¾ cup chicken broth
  ⅛ teaspoon saffron *or* ¼ teaspoon ground turmeric
  2 5-ounce cans *or* one 12½-ounce can chunk-style chicken, drained and flaked
  8 cherry tomatoes, halved

◆ **Stir** together rice mixture, *½ cup* of the broth, and the saffron in a large skillet. Cook and stir over medium heat until heated through. Stir in chicken and cherry tomatoes; cook about 2 minutes more or until heated through. If desired, stir in additional broth to make desired consistency. Makes 4 servings.

NUTRITION FACTS PER SERVING: 230 calories, 19 g protein, 23 g carbohydrate, 6 g fat, 39 mg cholesterol, 3 g dietary fiber, 487 mg sodium.

COOK RICE NOW—SERVE LATER

Be prepared for last-minute meals by precooking your rice, then stashing it in the refrigerator for up to 4 days, or in the freezer for up to 6 months.

Simply cook the rice according to package directions. Store the cooked rice in an airtight container or plastic freezer bag. To reheat chilled rice or frozen rice that has been thawed, in a saucepan combine the rice and 2 tablespoons of water for each cup of rice. Cover and heat over medium heat about 5 minutes or until rice is heated through.

CHICKEN AND FETTUCCINE WITH MUSTARD SAUCE

You can also substitute skinless, boneless chicken breasts cut lengthwise into 1-inch strips for the chicken tenderloins.

- 4 ounces refrigerated fettuccine
- 12 ounces chicken tenderloins
     Nonstick spray coating
- ½ cup sliced fresh mushrooms
- ½ cup fat-free dairy sour cream
- 2 teaspoons Dijon-style mustard
- ½ teaspoon dried thyme, crushed

◆ **Cook** pasta according to package directions, *except* use 4 cups lightly salted water; drain. Keep warm.

◆ **Meanwhile,** rinse chicken; pat dry. Spray an unheated large skillet with nonstick coating. Preheat skillet over medium heat. Add chicken and mushrooms; cook and stir for 6 to 8 minutes or until chicken is tender and no longer pink.

◆ **Stir** together sour cream, mustard, and thyme in a small bowl. Add sour cream mixture to skillet. Cook and stir until heated through (do not boil). Serve over pasta. Makes 4 servings.

NUTRITION FACTS PER SERVING: 240 calories, 22 g protein, 28 g carbohydrate, 3 g fat, 45 mg cholesterol, 0 g dietary fiber, 124 mg sodium.

CHICKEN AND FETA SALAD-STUFFED PITAS

To save time, thaw the chicken in the refrigerator overnight.

- ¾ cup loose-pack frozen peas
- 1 9-ounce package frozen chopped cooked chicken, thawed
- 1 medium tomato, chopped
- ¼ cup crumbled feta cheese (1 ounce)
- 2 green onions, sliced (¼ cup)
- ⅓ cup plain fat-free yogurt
- 1 teaspoon dried dillweed
- 4 pita bread rounds, halved crosswise
     Lettuce leaves

◆ **Rinse** peas under cold running water until thawed. Combine peas, chicken, tomato, feta cheese, and green onions. Stir in yogurt and dillweed; toss to combine. Line pita halves with lettuce. Spoon chicken mixture into pita halves. Serve immediately. Makes 4 servings.

NUTRITION FACTS PER SERVING: 349 calories, 28 g protein, 41 g carbohydrate, 7 g fat, 64 mg cholesterol, 2 g dietary fiber, 502 mg sodium.

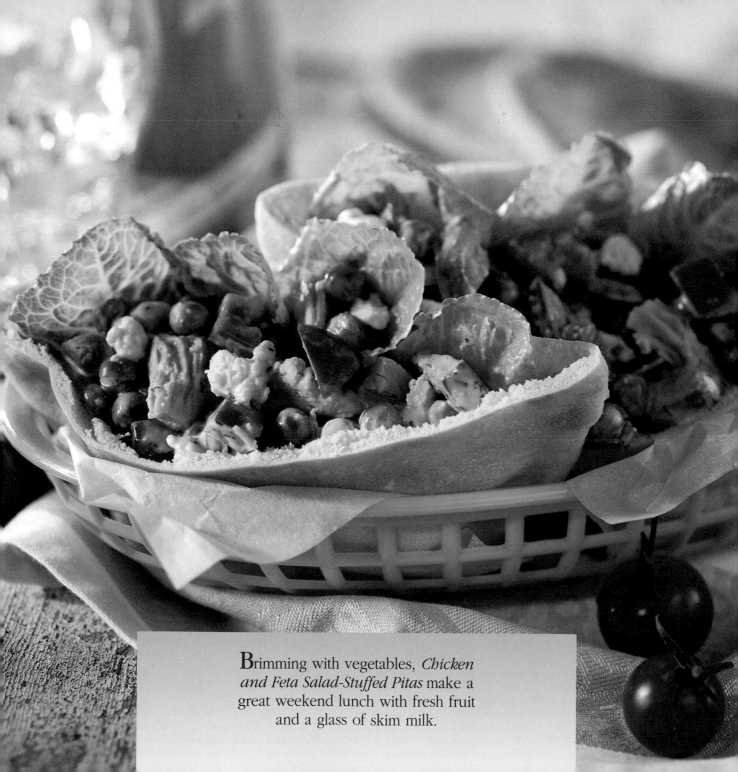

Brimming with vegetables, *Chicken and Feta Salad-Stuffed Pitas* make a great weekend lunch with fresh fruit and a glass of skim milk.

TURKEY WITH TROPICAL FRUIT SALSA

  4   turkey breast tenderloin steaks *or* medium skinless, boneless chicken breast halves
      (1 pound total)
  1   teaspoon olive oil *or* cooking oil
  1   15½-ounce can tropical fruit salad, drained and chopped
  2   tablespoons lime juice
  1   green onion, sliced (2 tablespoons)
  1   teaspoon chopped green chili peppers
  2   cups hot cooked rice (optional)

◆ **Set oven** to broil. Rinse turkey; pat dry. Place on unheated rack of a broiler pan. Brush with some of the oil. Broil 4 to 5 inches from heat for 7 minutes. Turn; brush with remaining oil. Sprinkle with salt and black pepper. Broil for 5 to 8 minutes more or until tender and no longer pink.

◆ **Meanwhile,** stir together drained and chopped fruit, lime juice, green onion, and chili peppers in a medium bowl. Serve with turkey over hot cooked rice, if desired. Makes 4 servings.

NUTRITION FACTS PER SERVING: 179 calories, 22 g protein, 15 g carbohydrate, 3 g fat, 50 mg cholesterol, 1 g dietary fiber, 118 mg sodium.

TURKEY SAUTÉ WITH MUSTARD SAUCE

  4   turkey breast tenderloin steaks (1 pound total)
      Nonstick spray coating
  ½   cup light dairy sour cream
  ¼   cup skim milk
  1   tablespoon honey
  2   teaspoons dry mustard
  ¼   teaspoon dried thyme, crushed
  2   tablespoons snipped fresh parsley
  2   cups hot cooked noodles

◆ **Rinse** turkey; pat dry. Spray an unheated large skillet with nonstick coating. Preheat skillet over medium heat. Add turkey; cook for 6 to 8 minutes or until tender and no longer pink, turning once. Transfer to a platter; cover to keep warm.

◆ **Remove** skillet from heat for 1 to 2 minutes to cool slightly. Add sour cream, milk, honey, dry mustard, thyme, and ⅛ teaspoon *pepper* to skillet; stir until combined. Cook and stir until heated through (do not boil). Stir in parsley. Spoon some of the sauce over the turkey. Pass remaining sauce. Serve with hot cooked noodles. Makes 4 servings.

NUTRITION FACTS PER SERVING: 280 calories, 28 g protein, 28 g carbohydrate, 6 g fat, 79 mg cholesterol, 2 g dietary fiber, 91 mg sodium.

SAUTÉED TURKEY WITH TOMATOES

Sauté turkey breasts, then top with tomato, basil, and low-fat mozzarella cheese, for an Italian-style dish with a low-fat American twist.

4	turkey breast tenderloin steaks (1 pound total)
⅛	teaspoon salt
	Nonstick spray coating
1	shallot, sliced
1	clove garlic, minced
4	thin tomato slices
1	tablespoon snipped fresh basil *or* 1 teaspoon dried basil, crushed
½	cup shredded reduced-fat mozzarella cheese (2 ounces)

◆ **Rinse** turkey; pat dry with paper towels. Sprinkle turkey with the salt. Spray an unheated large skillet with nonstick coating. Preheat the skillet over medium heat. Add turkey, shallot, and garlic; cook for 6 to 8 minutes or until turkey is tender and no longer pink, turning once.

◆ **Place** a tomato slice on each tenderloin steak in the skillet; sprinkle basil and shredded cheese over tomatoes. Cover skillet; heat about 2 minutes more or until the cheese melts. Makes 4 servings.

NUTRITION FACTS PER SERVING: 152 calories, 26 g protein, 3 g carbohydrate, 4 g fat, 55 mg cholesterol, 0 g dietary fiber, 190 mg sodium.

LEAN POULTRY CHOICES

Chicken and turkey are good choices for healthful eating, especially if you heed these simple, fat-fighting hints.

• Reduce fat in poultry by about 10 percent by removing the skin and pockets of fat under the skin.

• Be choosy about the type of meat you eat. Light meat, such as a breast, is leaner than dark meat, such as a thigh or leg.

• When a recipe calls for ground chicken or turkey, shop for the leanest meat you can find. To be assured you have the leanest ground chicken or turkey, ask the butcher to skin, bone, and grind chicken or turkey breast for you. Or, grind it yourself in a food grinder, using a coarse blade.

CURRIED CRAB SALAD

1   8½-ounce can unpeeled apricot halves, drained and cut in half
1   6-ounce package frozen crabmeat, thawed and drained
1   cup halved strawberries
¾   cup sliced celery
¼   cup light mayonnaise *or* salad dressing
¼   cup plain low-fat yogurt
1   to 2 tablespoons skim milk
½   teaspoon curry powder
4   cups purchased torn mixed salad greens

◆ **Combine** apricots, crabmeat, strawberries, and celery in a large mixing bowl.

◆ **For dressing,** stir together mayonnaise, yogurt, milk, and curry powder in a small mixing bowl. Line 3 individual serving plates with greens. Spoon some of the crab mixture onto each plate. Spoon on the dressing. Makes 3 servings.

NUTRITION FACTS PER SERVING: 153 calories, 10 g protein, 27 g carbohydrate, 1 g fat, 31 mg cholesterol, 3 g dietary fiber, 423 mg sodium.

CRUNCHY OVEN-FRIED FISH

1   pound fresh *or* frozen* orange roughy *or* other white fish fillets, ½ inch thick
¼   cup all-purpose flour
¼   teaspoon lemon-pepper seasoning
1   egg white
¼   cup fine dry bread crumbs
¼   cup cornmeal
1½   teaspoons finely shredded lemon peel
½   teaspoon dried basil, crushed
      Nonstick spray coating

◆ **Set oven** to 450°. Cut fish into serving-size pieces. Mix flour, lemon-pepper, and ¼ teaspoon *salt* in a shallow dish. Beat egg white until frothy; place in another shallow dish. Combine bread crumbs, cornmeal, lemon peel, and basil in a third shallow dish. Dip top of fillets into flour mixture; shake off any excess. Dip tops into egg white; coat with crumb mixture.

◆ **Spray** a shallow baking pan with nonstick coating. Place fillets in pan, coating side up; tuck under thin edges. Bake for 6 to 12 minutes or until fish flakes easily with a fork. Serves 4.

◆ ***Note:** Thaw fish, if frozen. To quick-thaw, see tip, *page 19.*

NUTRITION FACTS PER SERVING: 174 calories, 21 g protein, 18 g carbohydrate, 1 g fat, 43 mg cholesterol, 1 g dietary fiber, 333 mg sodium.

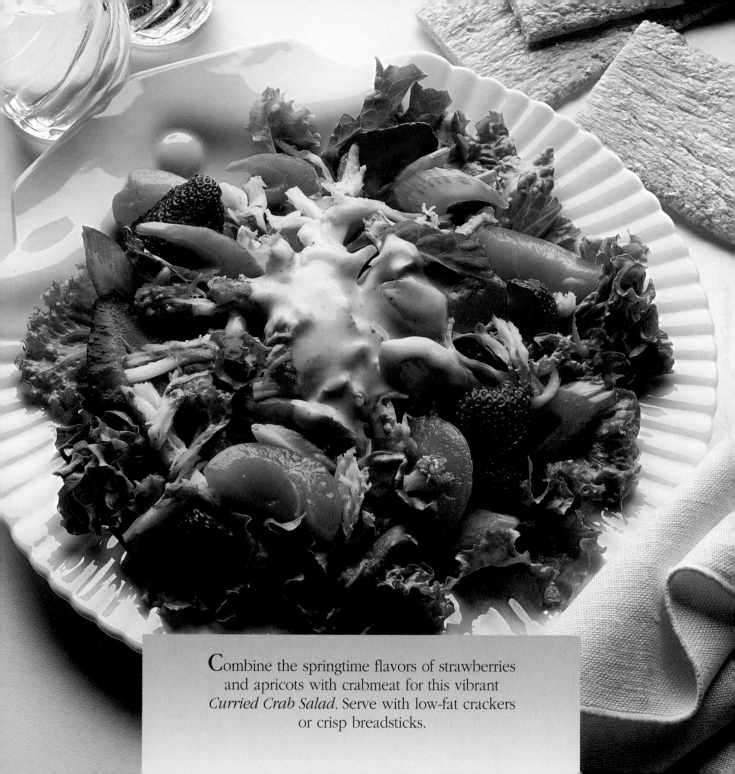

Combine the springtime flavors of strawberries and apricots with crabmeat for this vibrant *Curried Crab Salad*. Serve with low-fat crackers or crisp breadsticks.

FRUIT AND TUNA SALAD

Cooking for two? Turn to this colorful, simple salad, flavored with a luscious low-fat lemon-yogurt dressing.

  2 3½-ounce cans tuna (water-pack), drained
  1 cup halved seedless red grapes
  ½ cup purchased shredded cabbage with carrot (coleslaw mix)
  ⅓ cup lemon low-fat yogurt
  ⅔ cup purchased shredded cabbage with carrot (coleslaw mix)
  2 medium peaches, pitted and cut into wedges

◆ **Combine** tuna, *half* of the grapes, and the ½ cup shredded cabbage with carrot in a small bowl. Stir in the yogurt. Line 2 individual serving plates with remaining ⅔ cup shredded cabbage with carrot. Spoon tuna mixture on top. Serve with peach wedges and remaining grapes. Makes 2 servings.

NUTRITION FACTS PER SERVING: 253 calories, 25 g protein, 36 g carbohydrate, 2 g fat, 27 mg cholesterol, 4 g dietary fiber, 326 mg sodium.

LEMONY FISH FILLETS

Be sure to preheat your oven while you prepare the fish for baking. If using frozen fish, thaw the fillets overnight in the refrigerator or quick-thaw them in your microwave oven (see tip, opposite).

      Nonstick spray coating
  4 fresh *or* frozen skinless sole *or* flounder fillets, ¼ inch thick (12 ounces total)
  ½ teaspoon lemon-pepper seasoning
  1 Roma tomato, thinly sliced
  1 green onion, sliced (2 tablespoons)
  ½ teaspoon dried basil, crushed

◆ **Set oven** to 450°. Spray a 2-quart rectangular baking dish with nonstick coating. Place fish in baking dish. Sprinkle with lemon-pepper. Place tomato slices on top of fish. Sprinkle with green onion and basil. Bake for 4 to 6 minutes or until fish flakes easily with a fork. Makes 4 servings.

NUTRITION FACTS PER SERVING: 73 calories, 14 g protein, 1 g carbohydrate, 1 g fat, 40 mg cholesterol, 0 g dietary fiber, 199 mg sodium.

TARRAGON SHRIMP

1 9-ounce package refrigerated fettuccine
1 6-ounce package frozen pea pods
   Nonstick spray coating
12 ounces fresh *or* frozen,* peeled and deveined medium shrimp
½ teaspoon bottled minced garlic
1 cup evaporated skim milk
½ cup reduced-sodium chicken broth
1 tablespoon cornstarch
½ teaspoon dried tarragon *or* basil, crushed, *or* dried dillweed
   Cracked black pepper

◆ **Cook** pasta according to package directions; drain. Keep warm. Rinse pea pods under cold running water to separate; drain. Meanwhile, spray an unheated large skillet with nonstick coating. Preheat over medium heat. Add shrimp and garlic; cook and stir for 2 to 3 minutes or until shrimp turn pink. Remove from skillet.

◆ **Stir** together milk, chicken broth, cornstarch, tarragon, and ⅛ teaspoon *salt.* Add to skillet. Cook and stir until thickened and bubbly. Add pea pods. Cook and stir for 1 minute more. Add shrimp; heat through. Serve over pasta. Sprinkle with pepper. Makes 4 servings.

◆ ***Note:** Thaw shrimp, if frozen. To quick-thaw, see tip, *below.*

NUTRITION FACTS PER SERVING: 402 calories, 29 g protein, 64 g carbohydrate, 3 g fat, 133 mg cholesterol, 2 g dietary fiber, 374 mg sodium.

MICROWAVE QUICK-THAW FOR FISH AND SEAFOOD

Oops! Forget to defrost the fish or seafood for dinner? With a little help from your microwave oven, you can still get dinner to the table fast. Here's how.

Unwrap the frozen fish or seafood and place it in a microwave-safe dish. Cover and defrost on 30 percent power (medium-low) for the time listed *below.* Stir, turn, or separate the food halfway through defrosting time. Let food stand for 10 minutes to complete thawing.

• Fish, fillets (1 pound): 6 to 8 minutes
• Fish, steaks (1 pound): 6 to 8 minutes
• Shrimp, in shells (1 pound): 6 to 8 minutes
• Shrimp, peeled and deveined (1 pound): 7 to 9 minutes
• Crabmeat (6 ounces): 2½ to 3½ minutes

CHILI-SAUCED PASTA

    6 ounces refrigerated linguine
    1 14½-ounce can reduced-sodium stewed tomatoes
    1 medium green pepper, cut into thin, bite-size strips
    2 tablespoons reduced-sodium tomato paste
    1 tablespoon chili powder
    ¼ teaspoon garlic powder
    ¼ teaspoon ground cumin
    1 8-ounce can kidney beans, rinsed and drained
    2 teaspoons cornstarch

◆ **Cook** pasta according to package directions, *except* omit salt; drain. Keep warm. Meanwhile, mix *undrained* stewed tomatoes, green pepper, tomato paste, chili powder, garlic powder, cumin, and ¼ teaspoon *salt* in a saucepan. Bring to boiling; reduce heat. Simmer, covered, 3 minutes. Add beans.

◆ **Stir** together ¼ cup *water* and the cornstarch in bowl. Add to tomato mixture. Cook and stir until thickened and bubbly. Cook and stir 2 minutes more. Serve over pasta. Makes 3 servings.

NUTRITION FACTS PER SERVING: 322 calories, 15 g protein, 65 g carbohydrate, 2 g fat, 49 mg cholesterol, 10 g dietary fiber, 392 mg sodium.

CHEESE RAVIOLI WITH ZUCCHINI SAUCE

    1 9-ounce package reduced-fat refrigerated cheese-stuffed ravioli *or* tortellini
    1 15½-ounce can cannellini beans, rinsed and drained
    1 cup skim milk
    1 teaspoon cooking oil
    1 cup thinly sliced zucchini *and/or* yellow summer squash
    ½ cup red sweet pepper cut into thin, bite-size strips
    2 tablespoons grated Parmesan cheese
    1 teaspoon dried oregano, crushed

◆ **Cook** ravioli according to package directions, *except* use 4 cups water; drain. Keep warm. Meanwhile, place beans and milk in a food processor bowl or blender container. Cover and process or blend until smooth.

◆ **Heat** oil in large skillet over medium-high heat. Cook and stir zucchini and red pepper in skillet 2 to 3 minutes or until tender. Add bean mixture, Parmesan, oregano, and ⅛ teaspoon *black pepper.* Heat through. Toss with ravioli. Makes 4 servings.

NUTRITION FACTS PER SERVING: 325 calories, 22 g protein, 49 g carbohydrate, 8 g fat, 30 mg cholesterol, 5 g dietary fiber, 586 mg sodium.

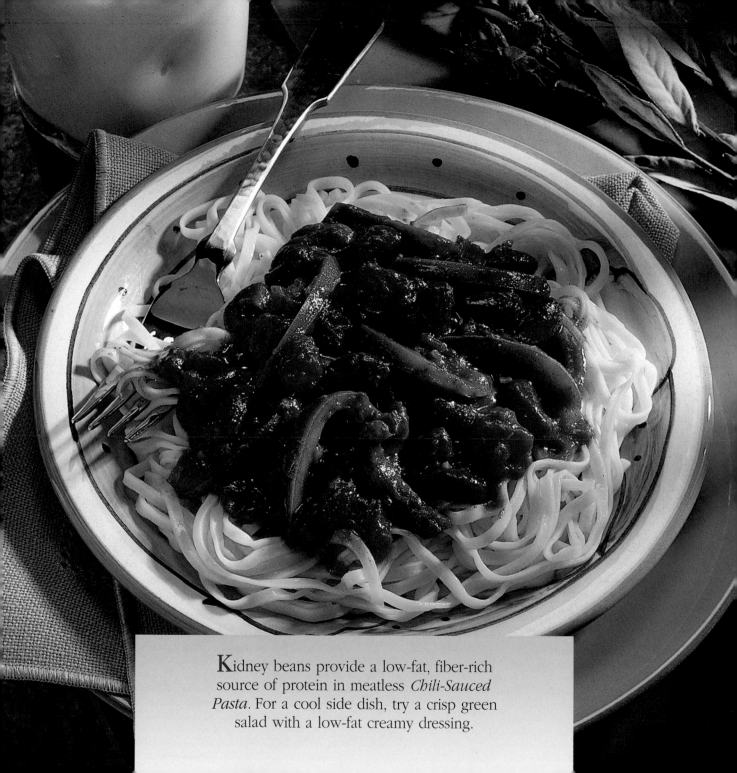

Kidney beans provide a low-fat, fiber-rich source of protein in meatless *Chili-Sauced Pasta*. For a cool side dish, try a crisp green salad with a low-fat creamy dressing.

MINT-GLAZED LAMB CHOPS

    1   teaspoon cornstarch
    3   tablespoons snipped fresh mint *or* 2 teaspoons dried mint, crushed
    1   tablespoon light corn syrup
    ½   teaspoon finely shredded lemon peel
    4   lamb leg sirloin chops, cut ¾ inch thick (about 1¼ pounds)

◆ **Set oven** to broil. For glaze, stir together ¼ cup *water* and the cornstarch in small saucepan. Add mint, corn syrup, lemon peel, and ¼ teaspoon *salt.* Cook and stir until thickened and bubbly. Cook and stir for 2 minutes more. Remove from heat.

◆ **Place** chops on the unheated rack of a broiler pan. Broil 3 inches from heat for 4 minutes. Brush chops with some of the glaze. Turn chops; broil for 4 to 5 minutes more for medium (160°) doneness, brushing occasionally with glaze. Makes 4 servings.

NUTRITION FACTS PER SERVING: 142 calories, 18 g protein, 5 g carbohydrate, 5 g fat, 57 mg cholesterol, 0 g dietary fiber, 181 mg sodium.

QUICK GREEK-STYLE BURRITOS

    ½   cup quick-cooking rice
    8   ounces 90% lean ground beef
    1   teaspoon bottled minced garlic
    ½   teaspoon dried oregano, crushed
    ½   teaspoon ground cumin
    ¼   to ½ teaspoon dried mint, crushed
    ¼   teaspoon salt
    ½   cup plain fat-free yogurt
    1   to 2 tablespoons skim milk (optional)
    8   6-inch flour tortillas
    1½ cups purchased torn mixed salad greens
        Several thin slices cucumber

◆ **Cook** rice according to package directions, *except* omit salt and margarine. Meanwhile, cook and stir beef and garlic in large skillet over medium-high heat until beef is brown; drain.

◆ **Stir** oregano, cumin, mint, salt, and ¼ teaspoon *pepper* into beef. Cook and stir for 1 minute. Remove from heat; stir in yogurt and rice. Stir in milk to thin sauce, if necessary.

◆ **Spoon** beef mixture onto centers of tortillas. Top with greens and cucumber slices. Roll up. Makes 4 servings.

NUTRITION FACTS PER SERVING: 333 calories, 18 g protein, 43 g carbohydrate, 9 g fat, 36 mg cholesterol, 0 g dietary fiber, 432 mg sodium.

CHUNKY POTATO CHOWDER

Serve this home-style soup with slices of crusty French bread. For heartier appetites, pair with a healthful sandwich (see tip, below, for suggestions).

    8 ounces 90% lean ground beef, ground raw turkey, *or* ground raw chicken
    2 cups skim milk
    2 cups frozen diced hash brown potatoes
    1 10¾-ounce can reduced-fat and reduced-sodium condensed cream of mushroom soup
    1 cup loose-pack frozen mixed vegetables
    2 tablespoons snipped dried tomato
    ½ teaspoon dried basil, crushed

◆ **Cook** and stir ground beef in a large saucepan over medium-high heat until brown; drain fat. Stir in milk, potatoes, condensed soup, and mixed vegetables. Bring to boiling. Stir in tomato bits and basil. Reduce the heat. Simmer, covered, about 5 minutes or until heated through. Makes 4 servings.

NUTRITION FACTS PER SERVING: 266 calories, 18 g protein, 33 g carbohydrate, 7 g fat, 39 mg cholesterol, 2 g dietary fiber, 309 mg sodium.

SMART SANDWICHES

Sandwiches are not only quick and easy to prepare, they can be healthful and satisfying, too. As you make sandwiches for your family, keep these nutritious ideas in mind.

• Use whole grain bread or rolls for increased fiber. Choose bread or rolls that list whole wheat flour (or another whole grain) as the first ingredient.

• Instead of mayonnaise, margarine, and butter, use mustard to boost flavor and decrease fat.

• Select low-fat luncheon meats. To reduce salt, cook and slice your own meats for sandwiches.

• Check out the growing selection of low-fat and nonfat cheeses. Use these instead of their higher-fat counterparts.

• Add plenty of texture, color, fiber, and flavor to your sandwich with fresh vegetables, such as lettuce, sweet pepper, red onion, cucumber, tomato, and shredded carrot.

ROAST BEEF AND PEPPERCORN PITAS

This quick, no-cook recipe offers a pita-pocketful of fresh, original flavors.

    3   cups purchased shredded cabbage with carrot (coleslaw mix)
    ¼   cup fat-free peppercorn ranch salad dressing
    3   tablespoons finely chopped onion
    8   ounces thinly sliced cooked roast beef
    4   pita bread rounds, halved crosswise
    ½   of a medium cucumber, thinly sliced

◆ **Combine** shredded cabbage with carrot, salad dressing, and onion in a medium bowl. Divide beef among pita halves. Add some of the cucumber slices and coleslaw mixture to each pita half. Serve immediately. Makes 4 servings.

NUTRITION FACTS PER SERVING: 334 calories, 24 g protein, 43 g carbohydrate, 7 g fat, 51 mg cholesterol, 2 g dietary fiber, 525 mg sodium.

GARDEN BEEF SALAD

Using purchased greens makes this standard, chef's-style salad extra simple. Fat-free dressing is the key ingredient for making it healthful. Pictured on pages 4–5.

    4   cups purchased torn mixed salad greens
    8   ounces thinly sliced cooked roast beef
    1   medium cucumber, thinly sliced
    1   small red onion, thinly sliced
    1   small yellow, red, *or* green sweet pepper, cut into bite-size strips
    ½   cup fat-free Italian *or* ranch salad dressing

◆ **Place** greens on a large serving platter. Arrange beef, cucumber, onion, and sweet pepper on top. Serve with dressing. Makes 4 servings.

NUTRITION FACTS PER SERVING: 187 calories, 19 g protein, 12 g carbohydrate, 6 g fat, 54 mg cholesterol, 2 g dietary fiber, 337 mg sodium.

HAM AND ASPARAGUS OMELETS

Enjoy these savory omelets any time of day. If you'd like, you can replace the whole eggs and egg whites with 1 cup refrigerated or thawed frozen egg substitute.

	Nonstick spray coating
1½	cups loose-pack frozen cut asparagus
1	cup chopped reduced-fat, reduced-sodium fully cooked ham
⅓	cup fat-free dairy sour cream
4	egg whites
2	eggs
⅛	teaspoon garlic powder
2	tablespoons fat-free dairy sour cream

◆ **Spray** an unheated 8-inch skillet and an unheated 10-inch nonstick skillet with flared sides with nonstick coating. Preheat the 8-inch skillet over medium heat. Add asparagus; cook and stir for 3 minutes. Reduce heat to low. Add ham and the ⅓ cup sour cream; heat through. Set aside.

◆ **Beat** together egg whites, eggs, garlic powder, 1 tablespoon *water* and ⅛ teaspoon *pepper.* Preheat 10-inch skillet over medium heat. Add *half* of egg mixture; lift and tilt skillet to spread mixture. As mixture sets, run a spatula around edge of skillet, lifting mixture as necessary to let uncooked portion flow underneath. When the egg mixture is set but still shiny, remove from heat. Spoon *half* of asparagus mixture across center of omelet. Fold the sides over; transfer to platter.

◆ **Repeat** with remaining egg and asparagus mixtures. Halve omelets to serve. Top each with some of the 2 tablespoons sour cream. Makes 4 servings.

NUTRITION FACTS PER SERVING: 131 calories, 16 g protein, 8 g carbohydrate, 4 g fat, 122 mg cholesterol, 1 g dietary fiber, 494 mg sodium.

ENJOY A GOOD EGG WITH EGG SUBSTITUTES

Thanks to modern technology, there are a variety of refrigerated and frozen egg substitutes that allow you to easily enjoy egg dishes without worrying about cholesterol. These products, based mostly on egg whites, contain less fat than whole eggs, and no cholesterol. To adapt recipes for yeast breads, muffins, cakes, cookies, sauces, egg casseroles, custards, and puddings, use ¼ cup of egg substitute for each large whole egg. If a recipe calls for an egg yolk, use 2 tablespoons egg substitute instead. This product is not recommended for cream puffs or popovers.

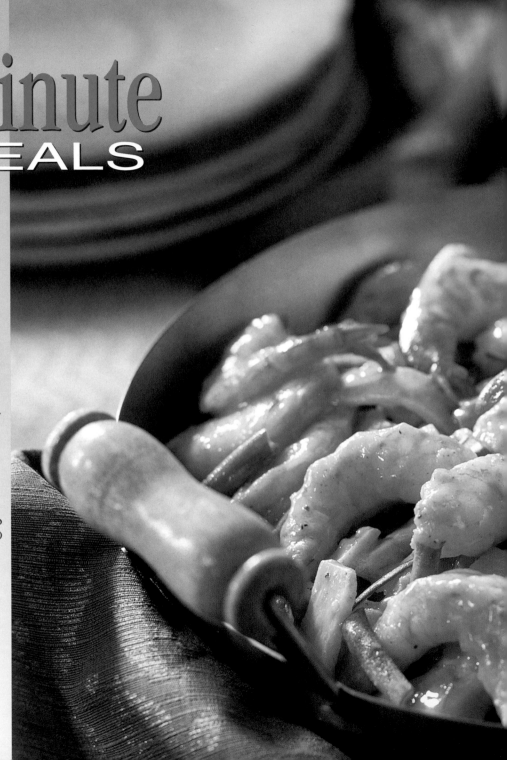

20-Minute
MEALS

Only 20 minutes until dinner, and you want a meal that's guilt free, fuss free, *and* full flavored? No problem—just turn to these pages for today's tasty solutions to life's little cooking challenges. You'll be enjoying a healthful home-cooked meal in minutes.

Sunshine Shrimp
(see recipe, *page 50*)

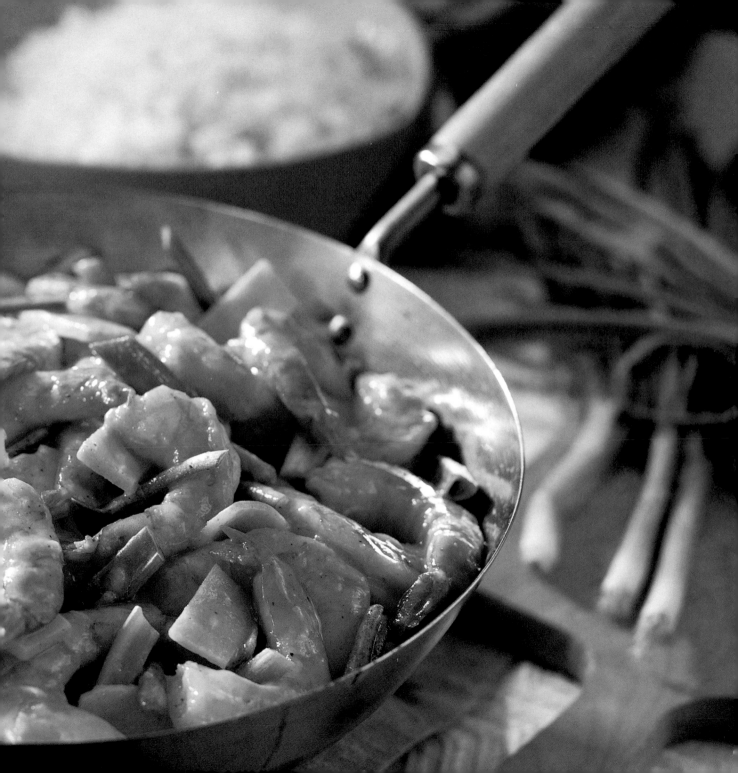

CHICKEN PARMIGIANA

To skim the fat from this Italian favorite, use nonstick spray coating to brown the crumb-coated chicken pieces, and skip the traditional mozzarella cheese topping.

- ¼ cup fine dry bread crumbs
- 2 tablespoons grated Parmesan cheese
- 4 small skinless, boneless chicken breast halves (12 ounces total)
- 2 tablespoons skim milk
  Nonstick spray coating
- 1 14½-ounce can stewed tomatoes
- 2 teaspoons cornstarch
- ½ teaspoon dried Italian seasoning, crushed
- 1 tablespoon grated Parmesan cheese

♦ **Combine** bread crumbs and the 2 tablespoons Parmesan cheese in a shallow dish or on a sheet of waxed paper.

♦ **Rinse** chicken; pat dry with paper towels. Brush chicken with milk. Coat chicken with crumb mixture.

♦ **Spray** an unheated large skillet with nonstick coating. Preheat skillet over medium heat. Add chicken; cook for 8 to 10 minutes or until tender and no longer pink, turning the pieces occasionally to brown evenly on all sides. Transfer to a platter; cover to keep warm. Wipe skillet with paper towels.

♦ **Combine** *undrained* stewed tomatoes, cornstarch, and Italian seasoning in the same skillet. Cook and stir until thickened and bubbly. Cook and stir for 2 minutes more.

♦ **Spoon** tomato mixture over chicken. Sprinkle with the 1 tablespoon Parmesan cheese. Makes 4 servings.

NUTRITION FACTS PER SERVING: 177 calories, 20 g protein, 14 g carbohydrate, 4 g fat, 48 mg cholesterol, 0 g dietary fiber, 499 mg sodium.

CHICKEN À LA KING

Healthful cooking does not have to mean forgoing traditional favorites. In this classic, vegetables are cooked in broth instead of oil to cut the fat.

1½ cups sliced fresh mushrooms *or* one 4½-ounce jar sliced mushrooms, drained
1   cup reduced-sodium chicken broth
1   small green *or* red sweet pepper, chopped (½ cup)
1   12-ounce can evaporated skim *or* low-fat milk
⅓   cup all-purpose flour
1½ cups cubed cooked chicken *or* turkey (about 8 ounces)
¼   cup diced pimiento
¼   cup dry sherry *or* dry white wine
1   teaspoon Worcestershire sauce
⅛   teaspoon black pepper
    Toast Points (see recipe, *below*) *or* 4 English muffins, split and toasted

◆ **Stir** together the fresh mushrooms (if using), chicken broth, and sweet pepper in a medium saucepan. Bring to boiling; reduce heat. Simmer, covered, for 2 minutes or until the vegetables are tender. Do not drain.

◆ **Meanwhile,** gradually stir the milk into the flour until smooth. Stir into vegetable mixture. Cook and stir over high heat until thickened and bubbly. Cook and stir for 1 minute more. Stir in canned mushrooms (if using), chicken, pimiento, sherry, Worcestershire sauce, and black pepper. Heat through.

◆ **To serve,** arrange Toast Points on individual serving plates. Spoon chicken mixture over toast. Makes 4 servings.

◆ **Toast Points:** Toast 4 slices of whole wheat or white bread. Cut each slice diagonally in half. Cut each half slice in half again to form 4 triangles from each slice of bread.

NUTRITION FACTS PER SERVING: 348 calories, 28 g protein, 37 g carbohydrate, 8 g fat, 58 mg cholesterol, 4 g dietary fiber, 457 mg sodium.

CHICKEN WITH CHERRY SAUCE

  4 small skinless, boneless chicken breast halves (12 ounces total)
      Ground nutmeg
⅓ cup reduced-sodium chicken broth
⅓ cup unsweetened pineapple juice
  2 teaspoons cornstarch
  1 teaspoon brown sugar
¼ cup dried tart red cherries *or* light raisins, coarsely chopped

◆ **Set oven** to broil. Rinse chicken; pat dry with paper towels. Sprinkle lightly with nutmeg. Place chicken, boned side up, on the unheated rack of broiler pan. Broil 4 to 5 inches from the heat for 7 minutes. Turn chicken; broil for 5 to 8 minutes more or until tender and no longer pink.

◆ **Meanwhile, for sauce,** combine chicken broth, pineapple juice, cornstarch, brown sugar, and dash *pepper* in a small saucepan. Cook and stir over medium heat until thickened and bubbly. Stir in cherries. Cook and stir for 2 minutes more. Serve cherry sauce over chicken. Makes 4 servings.

NUTRITION FACTS PER SERVING: 138 calories, 17 g protein, 11 g carbohydrate, 2 g fat, 45 mg cholesterol, 0 g dietary fiber, 94 mg sodium.

REMODELING YOUR FAVORITE RECIPES TO REDUCE FAT

Increase your odds for good health with these simple, fat-fighting strategies:

• Choose cooking techniques that reduce, rather than add, fat. Broil, grill, steam, roast, poach, or micro-cook.

• Use nonstick spray coating instead of oil when you sauté and stir-fry. Or, cook foods in a small amount of broth or water rather than sautéing them in oil.

• Select lean cuts of meat, then trim visible fat. Plan on 4 ounces (3 ounces cooked) of meat per serving.

• Remove poultry skin before or after cooking.

• Cook soups and stews ahead, then chill and remove fat.

• Top off salads with nonfat or low-fat salad dressings. Or, season them with herbs and flavored vinegar.

• Substitute! Whenever possible, use lower-fat versions of the ingredients you would normally use to prepare recipes.

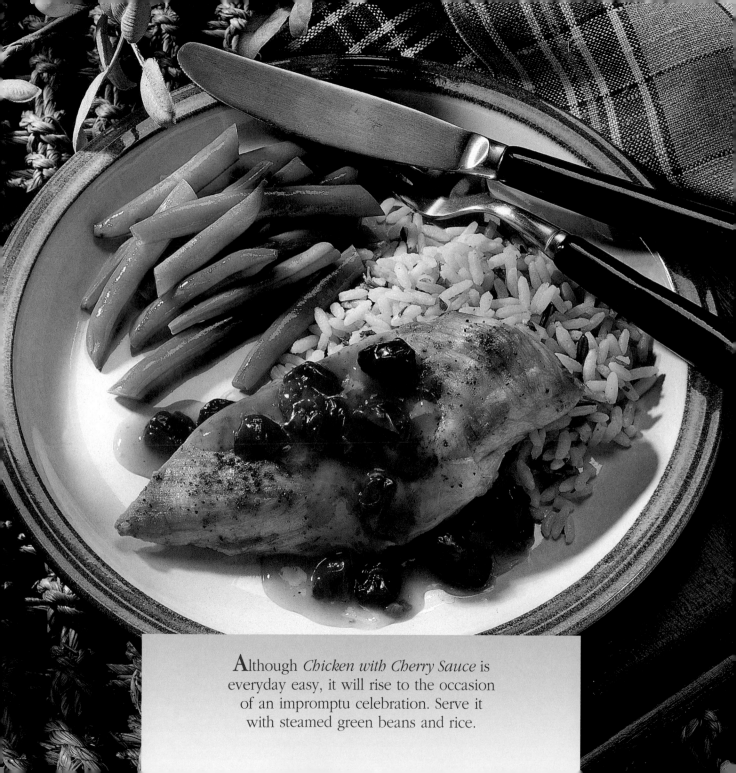

Although *Chicken with Cherry Sauce* is
everyday easy, it will rise to the occasion
of an impromptu celebration. Serve it
with steamed green beans and rice.

QUICK CHICKEN ORIENTAL

To skip the chopping step, this timesaving stir-fry calls on precut fresh vegetables for stir-frying, found in the produce section of the supermarket, or a frozen vegetable combination.

12 ounces skinless, boneless chicken breast halves *or* turkey breast tenderloins
⅓ cup orange juice
2 tablespoons light soy sauce
2 teaspoons cornstarch
1 teaspoon brown sugar
½ teaspoon ground ginger
    Nonstick spray coating
1 16-ounce package fresh cut-up Oriental stir-fry vegetables *or* one 16-ounce package
     loose-pack frozen broccoli, red peppers, bamboo shoots, and straw mushrooms
1 tablespoon cooking oil
3 cups hot cooked rice

◆ **Rinse** chicken or turkey; pat dry with paper towels. Cut into thin, bite-size strips.

◆ **For sauce,** stir together orange juice, soy sauce, cornstarch, brown sugar, and ginger in a small bowl; set aside.

◆ **Spray** an unheated wok or large skillet with nonstick coating. Preheat over medium heat. Add Oriental vegetables; stir-fry for 2 to 3 minutes for fresh vegetables (4 to 5 minutes for frozen vegetables) or until crisp-tender. Remove from wok.

◆ **Pour** oil into hot wok. Add the chicken; stir-fry for 2 to 3 minutes or until chicken is tender and no longer pink. Push chicken from center of wok. Stir sauce; pour into center of wok. Cook and stir until thickened and bubbly.

◆ **Return** the cooked vegetables to the wok. Stir to coat all ingredients with sauce. Cook and stir about 1 minute more or until heated through. Serve with hot cooked rice. Makes 4 servings.

NUTRITION FACTS PER SERVING: 338 calories, 21 g protein, 46 g carbohydrate, 7 g fat, 45 mg cholesterol, 0 g dietary fiber, 328 mg sodium.

LINGUINE WITH CHICKEN AND CLAM SAUCE

  8 ounces packaged dried linguine *or* fettuccine
     Nonstick spray coating
  8 ounces ground raw chicken *or* turkey
  1 medium onion, chopped (½ cup)
  2 cloves garlic, minced
  ½ teaspoon dried basil, crushed
  ¼ cup all-purpose flour
1¼ cups reduced-sodium chicken broth
  ¾ cup evaporated skim milk
  1 10-ounce can whole baby clams, drained
  ¼ cup snipped fresh parsley
  ¼ cup dry white wine

◆ **Cook** pasta according to package directions, *except* omit salt and oil; drain. Keep warm.

◆ **Meanwhile,** spray unheated large saucepan with nonstick coating. Preheat saucepan over medium heat. Add chicken, onion, garlic, basil, ⅛ teaspoon *salt,* and ⅛ teaspoon *pepper;* cook and stir until chicken is no longer pink and onion is tender. Stir in flour. Add broth and milk. Cook and stir until thickened and bubbly. Cook and stir for 1 minute more. Stir in clams, parsley, and wine; heat through. Serve over pasta. Makes 4 servings.

NUTRITION FACTS PER SERVING: 407 calories, 26 g protein, 60 g carbohydrate, 5 g fat, 43 mg cholesterol, 1 g dietary fiber, 301 mg sodium.

PASTA PRESTO

Next time you cook pasta, throw a little extra in the pot. You can refrigerate or freeze it for another meal.

Store cooked pasta in airtight containers in the refrigerator for 3 to 5 days. If possible, store pasta and sauce separately. To reheat, drop pasta in boiling water for a few seconds and drain.

Or, to freeze cooked pasta for up to 2 weeks, cool the pasta slightly, then drizzle with a little olive oil or cooking oil and toss gently. Spoon into airtight containers or freezer bags.

Defrost a bag of frozen pasta in a colander in the sink by running tepid water over it. Or, drop the contents of the bag or container into boiling water. Thawing and warming time depends on the amount of pasta; plan on cooking frozen pasta about 2 minutes for small amounts.

CHICKEN WITH SALSA COUSCOUS

Couscous, a ricelike staple of North African cooking, is made from semolina wheat and shaped like tiny beads. Look for couscous near the rice or pasta in your supermarket.

  4 small skinless, boneless chicken breast halves (12 ounces total)
1⅓ cups chunky salsa
 ½ cup water
 ⅔ cup couscous
     Parsley sprigs (optional)
     Snipped fresh parsley (optional)

◆ **Set oven** to broil. Rinse chicken; pat dry with paper towels. Place chicken breast halves, boned side up, on the unheated rack of a broiler pan. Broil 4 to 5 inches from the heat for 7 minutes. Turn and broil for 5 to 8 minutes more or until chicken is tender and no longer pink.

◆ **Meanwhile,** heat salsa and water to boiling in a small saucepan; stir in couscous. Cover; remove from heat and let stand for 5 minutes.

◆ **Spoon** hot couscous onto 4 individual serving plates. Diagonally slice hot cooked chicken pieces; place on couscous. Garnish with a parsley sprig and snipped fresh parsley, if desired. Makes 4 servings.

NUTRITION FACTS PER SERVING: 233 calories, 21 g protein, 29 g carbohydrate, 4 g fat, 45 mg cholesterol, 5 g dietary fiber, 340 mg sodium.

FAST FIX-UPS WITH CHICKEN BREASTS

Keep a package of skinless, boneless chicken breasts stashed in your freezer, and you can spin off salads, stir-fries, and other healthy entrées—fast! For starters, try these flavorful fixes.

• *Speedy Chicken Caesar Salad:* Toss stir-fried chicken strips with precut salad greens and fat-free Caesar dressing. Sprinkle some grated Parmesan cheese over top.

• *Italian Chicken Stir-Fry:* Stir-fry chicken with reduced-fat Italian salad dressing. Then stir-fry frozen mixed vegetables; combine with chicken. Serve over quick-cooked brown rice.

• *Pepper-Cheese Chicken Sandwiches:* Serve broiled chicken breasts in French rolls, topped with slices of reduced-fat mozzarella cheese and roasted red peppers.

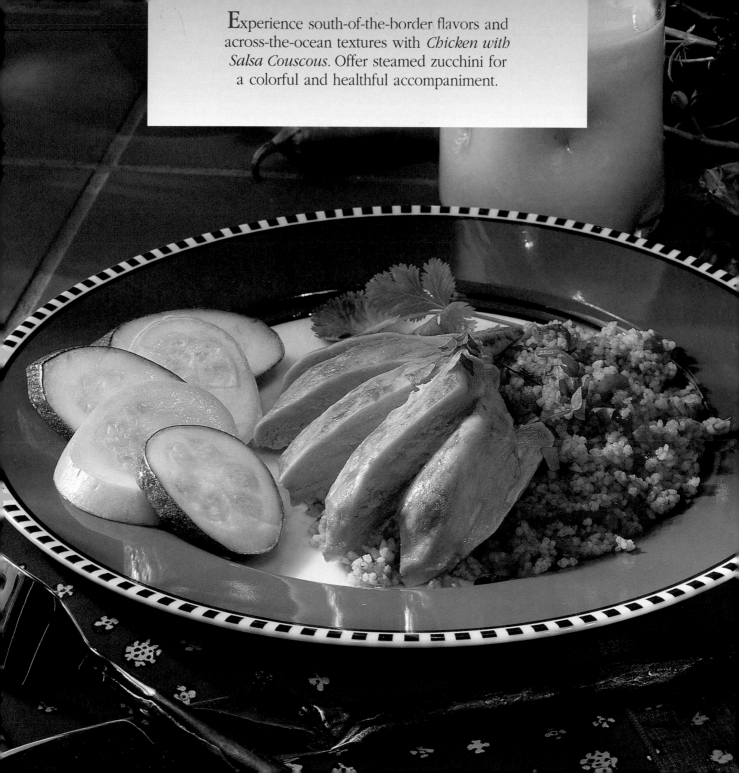

Experience south-of-the-border flavors and across-the-ocean textures with *Chicken with Salsa Couscous*. Offer steamed zucchini for a colorful and healthful accompaniment.

CHICKEN BULGUR SKILLET

Skip a step! Cook the bulgur, which lends a delicate nutty flavor to this dish, in the skillet along with the vegetables.

   8 ounces skinless, boneless chicken breast halves
      Nonstick spray coating
1½ cups frozen pepper stir-fry vegetables (yellow, green, and red sweet peppers and onions)
 ¾ cup reduced-sodium chicken broth
 ¾ cup water
 ½ cup quick-cooking rice
 ⅓ cup bulgur
   1 teaspoon dried Italian seasoning, crushed
 ⅛ teaspoon black pepper
   1 large zucchini *or* yellow summer squash, halved lengthwise and thinly sliced
 ½ cup shredded reduced-fat mozzarella cheese (2 ounces)

◆ **Rinse** chicken; pat dry with paper towels. Cut into thin, bite-size strips. Spray an unheated large skillet with nonstick coating. Preheat over medium heat. Add chicken; cook and stir about 3 minutes or until chicken is tender and no longer pink. Remove from skillet; set aside.

◆ **Add** stir-fry vegetables, chicken broth, water, *uncooked* rice, bulgur, Italian seasoning, and black pepper to skillet. Bring to boiling; reduce heat. Simmer, covered, for 4 minutes. Add zucchini; cook, uncovered, for 3 to 5 minutes more or until bulgur and zucchini are tender. Stir in chicken; heat through. Remove from heat.

◆ **Sprinkle** with the shredded cheese. Cover and let stand for 1 to 2 minutes or until cheese is melted. Makes 4 servings.

NUTRITION FACTS PER SERVING: 211 calories, 18 g protein, 25 g carbohydrate, 5 g fat, 38 mg cholesterol, 3 g dietary fiber, 228 mg sodium.

LEMON-PEPPER CHICKEN WITH MUSHROOM SAUCE

Evaporated skim milk enriches the broth-based sauce without adding extra fat. Be sure to start the noodles before you cook the chicken.

4	medium skinless, boneless chicken breast halves (1 pound total)
¼	teaspoon lemon-pepper seasoning
	Nonstick spray coating
2	cups sliced fresh mushrooms
½	cup reduced-sodium chicken broth
½	cup evaporated skim milk
1	tablespoon cornstarch
1	tablespoon Dijon-style mustard
2	cups hot cooked fine noodles
1	green onion, sliced (2 tablespoons)

◆ **Rinse** chicken; pat dry with paper towels. Sprinkle chicken with lemon-pepper seasoning. Spray an unheated large skillet with nonstick coating. Preheat over medium heat. Add chicken; cook for 8 to 10 minutes or until chicken is tender and no longer pink, turning once. Remove chicken from skillet; cover and keep warm.

◆ **Add** mushrooms to skillet; cook and stir for 2 minutes. Combine chicken broth, evaporated skim milk, cornstarch, and mustard in a small bowl; add to skillet. Cook and stir until thickened and bubbly; cook and stir for 2 minutes more.

◆ **Arrange** chicken on top of the noodles. Spoon sauce over all. Sprinkle with green onion. Makes 4 servings.

NUTRITION FACTS PER SERVING: 241 calories, 23 g protein, 26 g carbohydrate, 4 g fat, 71 mg cholesterol, 2 g dietary fiber, 323 mg sodium.

ITALIAN TURKEY BURGERS

*Don't hurry these savory burgers too much! They must cook the full 10 minutes—
until no pink remains.*

  1   egg white
  1   tablespoon catsup
  ½   teaspoon dried Italian seasoning, crushed
  ⅛   teaspoon salt
  ⅛   teaspoon pepper
  1   small zucchini, coarsely shredded (1 cup)
  ¼   cup fine dry bread crumbs
  1   pound ground raw turkey breast *or* ground raw chicken breast
  6   thin slices reduced-fat mozzarella cheese (3 ounces)
  6   whole wheat buns, split

◆ **Set oven** to broil. Meanwhile, combine the egg white, catsup, Italian seasoning, salt, and pepper in a large mixing bowl. Stir in zucchini and bread crumbs. Add turkey; mix well. Shape into six ½-inch-thick patties.

◆ **Place** the patties on the unheated rack of a broiler pan. Broil 3 inches from the heat about 10 minutes or until no longer pink, turning once.* Top each patty with a slice of cheese. Broil for 30 seconds more or until cheese begins to melt. Serve on buns. Makes 6 servings.

◆ ***Note:** If desired, add the split buns to the broiler pan and toast during the last 1 to 1½ minutes of broiling time.

NUTRITION FACTS PER SERVING: 251 calories, 20 g protein, 26 g carbohydrate, 8 g fat, 32 mg cholesterol, 3 g dietary fiber, 413 mg sodium.

CHICKEN AND TROPICAL FRUIT PLATE

Instead of peeling the kiwi fruit, rub the brown skin with a clean cloth to remove the excess fuzz.

    Lettuce leaves
 2 cups refrigerated mango* *or* papaya slices, drained
 2 kiwi fruit, peeled and sliced
 1 cup seedless red *or* green grapes
 8 ounces sliced fully cooked chicken luncheon meat
 ½ cup plain low-fat yogurt
 1 tablespoon honey
 ½ teaspoon poppy seed
    Melba toast

◆ **Line** 4 individual serving plates with lettuce. Arrange mango, kiwi fruit, and grapes on the plates. Roll up chicken luncheon meat and arrange on plates next to fruit.

◆ **For dressing,** stir together the yogurt, honey, and poppy seed in a small bowl. Drizzle over fruit and chicken. Serve with melba toast. Makes 4 servings.

◆ ***Note:** If desired, substitute 2 fresh bananas, sliced, and 1 large apple, cut into chunks, for the mango.

NUTRITION FACTS PER SERVING: 276 calories, 15 g protein, 36 g carbohydrate, 9 g fat, 43 mg cholesterol, 4 g dietary fiber, 449 mg sodium.

SALAD DRESSING SMARTS

You'll find an impressive array of salad dressings and mayonnaise on the shelves of your supermarket. Next to the regular dressings and mayonnaise are low-calorie, low-fat, nonfat, no-cholesterol, and low-cholesterol products. Check the nutrition labels—at a glance, you can compare calories, fat, cholesterol, and sodium, and then choose the dressing or mayonnaise that best fits your needs.

TURKEY MARSALA

Sometimes called the "filet mignon" of the turkey, turkey breast tenderloins are skinless, boneless cuts of turkey from the eye of the breast.

  4 turkey breast tenderloin steaks (1 pound total)
     Nonstick spray coating
  2 cloves garlic, minced
  ½ cup reduced-sodium chicken broth
  ¼ cup dry marsala
  1 tablespoon lemon juice
  ½ teaspoon salt-free seasoning blend
  ⅛ teaspoon pepper
  2 tablespoons snipped fresh parsley
     Steamed vegetables (optional)

◆ **Rinse** turkey; pat dry with paper towels. Spray an unheated large skillet with nonstick coating. Preheat skillet over medium heat. Add turkey steaks and garlic; cook for 6 to 8 minutes or until turkey is tender and no longer pink, turning once. Transfer to a serving platter; cover to keep warm.

◆ **For sauce,** add broth, wine, lemon juice, seasoning blend, and pepper to the skillet; mix well. Bring to boiling; boil gently, uncovered, about 4 minutes or until reduced to ¼ *cup* liquid. Stir in the parsley. Serve turkey over steamed vegetables, if desired. Spoon the sauce over turkey. Makes 4 servings.

NUTRITION FACTS PER SERVING: 139 calories, 22 g protein, 2 g carbohydrate, 3 g fat, 50 mg cholesterol, 0 g dietary fiber, 56 mg sodium.

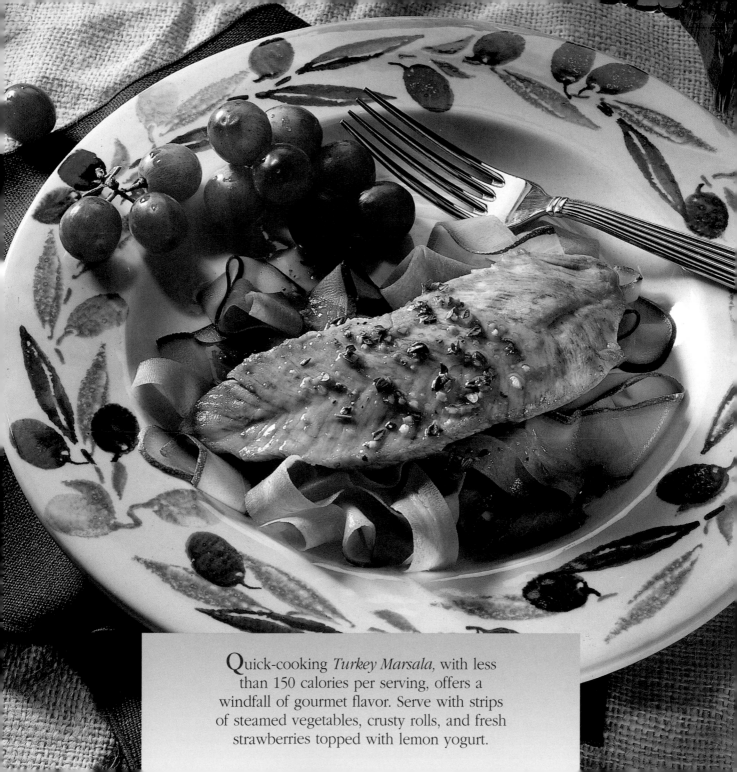

Quick-cooking *Turkey Marsala,* with less than 150 calories per serving, offers a windfall of gourmet flavor. Serve with strips of steamed vegetables, crusty rolls, and fresh strawberries topped with lemon yogurt.

WALDORF TURKEY SALAD WITH CANTALOUPE

No need to wait for holiday leftovers to enjoy turkey in your salads. Purchase precooked turkey breast or cook turkey breast or turkey breast tenderloins any time of year.

1 cup vanilla low-fat yogurt
¼ teaspoon apple pie spice *or* pumpkin pie spice
Dash salt
1 cup chopped pear *or* apple
1 teaspoon lemon juice
2 cups chopped cooked turkey *or* chicken (10 ounces)
1 cup halved seedless red *or* green grapes
1 stalk celery, chopped (½ cup)
1 green onion, sliced (2 tablespoons)
1 small cantaloupe
Red-tip leaf lettuce
¼ cup slivered almonds, toasted

◆ **For dressing,** combine yogurt, apple pie spice, and salt in a small mixing bowl. Set aside.

◆ **Toss** pear with lemon juice in a medium mixing bowl. Stir in turkey, grapes, celery, and green onion. Pour dressing over turkey mixture. Toss lightly to coat.

◆ **Cut** cantaloupe into 4 wedges. Remove seeds and, if desired, the rind. Line 4 individual serving plates with lettuce. Place cantaloupe wedges on the lettuce-lined plates. Stir toasted almonds into turkey mixture. Spoon onto cantaloupe wedges. Makes 4 servings.

NUTRITION FACTS PER SERVING: 340 calories, 26 g protein, 36 g carbohydrate, 12 g fat, 71 mg cholesterol, 4 g dietary fiber, 143 mg sodium.

NUTRITIOUS PASTA

The word pasta means paste, and most pasta starts with a paste of wheat flour and water. Except for egg noodles, pasta does not contain eggs; the creamy golden color comes from the durum wheat that is used.

A 1-cup serving of cooked pasta contains 190 calories, about 1 gram of fat, and no cholesterol. A complex carbohydrate, pasta is a good source of protein, as well as thiamin, riboflavin, niacin, and iron.

PASTA PRIMAVERA WITH SALMON

Skim milk and lower-fat sour cream lighten up the rich-tasting salmon sauce that's tossed with tender fettuccine and vegetables. Pictured on the cover.

1	16-ounce package loose-pack frozen broccoli, cauliflower, and red peppers
1	9-ounce package refrigerated plain *or* herbed fettuccine *or* linguine
1	7¾-ounce can salmon
1	tablespoon margarine *or* butter
1½	cups packaged presliced fresh mushrooms (4 ounces)
1	teaspoon bottled minced garlic
1	tablespoon cornstarch
½	teaspoon dried tarragon, crushed
1¼	cups skim milk
½	cup light dairy sour cream
¼	cup purchased shredded Parmesan *or* Romano cheese (1 ounce)
1	teaspoon Dijon-style mustard

◆ **Cook** vegetables and pasta separately according to package directions, *except* use 4 cups water when cooking pasta; drain. Keep warm. Meanwhile, drain salmon. Remove skin and bones; break salmon into large pieces.

◆ **Heat** margarine in a large skillet over medium-high heat until melted. Cook and stir mushrooms and garlic in skillet for 4 minutes. Reduce heat to medium. Stir in cornstarch and tarragon. Add milk; cook and stir until thickened and bubbly. Stir in sour cream, *half* of the Parmesan cheese, and the mustard. Gently stir in salmon; heat through.

◆ **To serve,** toss salmon mixture with vegetables and pasta. Transfer to a serving platter. Sprinkle with the remaining Parmesan cheese. Serve immediately. Makes 4 servings.

NUTRITION FACTS PER SERVING: 495 calories, 30 g protein, 68 g carbohydrate, 11 g fat, 40 mg cholesterol, 4 g dietary fiber, 541 mg sodium.

CHICKEN AND ORANGE STIR-FRY

This recipe cuts down on cutting and chopping chores with frozen stir-fry vegetables and canned mandarin oranges.

    2 cups frozen pepper stir-fry vegetables (yellow, green, and red sweet peppers and onions)
    1 11-ounce can mandarin oranges *or* one 8-ounce can pineapple chunks (juice pack)
    ¼ cup mango chutney, snipped
    ¼ cup orange juice
    3 tablespoons light soy sauce
    2 teaspoons cornstarch
    1 teaspoon bottled minced garlic
    ¼ teaspoon ground ginger
    8 ounces skinless, boneless chicken breast halves
       Nonstick spray coating
    2 cups hot cooked rice *or* couscous
       Green onion, cut into thin strips (optional)

◆ **Place** stir-fry vegetables in a colander. Rinse under cold running water until thawed; drain. Meanwhile, drain oranges, reserving *2 tablespoons* of the liquid. Stir together the reserved liquid, chutney, orange juice, soy sauce, cornstarch, garlic, and ginger in a small bowl. Set aside.

◆ **Rinse** chicken; pat dry with paper towels. Cut into bite-size strips.

◆ **Spray** an unheated wok or large skillet with nonstick coating. Preheat over medium heat. Add chicken; stir-fry about 3 minutes or until chicken is tender and no longer pink. Push chicken from center of wok.

◆ **Stir** soy sauce mixture; pour into center of wok. Cook and stir until thickened and bubbly. Add stir-fry vegetables. Stir to coat all ingredients with sauce. Cook, covered, for 2 minutes more. Gently stir in oranges; heat through. Serve with hot cooked rice. Garnish with thin strips of green onion, if desired. Makes 4 servings.

NUTRITION FACTS PER SERVING: 283 calories, 15 g protein, 50 g carbohydrate, 2 g fat, 30 mg cholesterol, 1 g dietary fiber, 446 mg sodium.

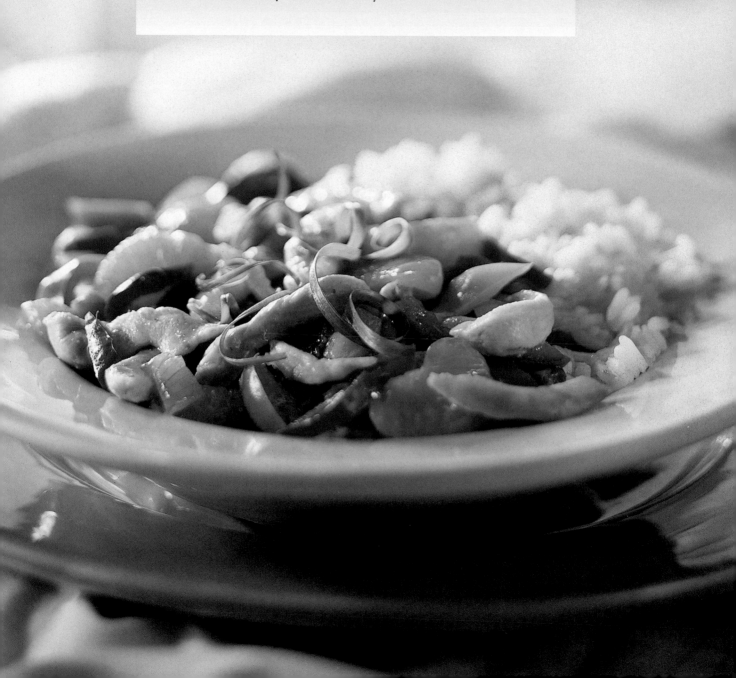

Sizzling in just 20 minutes, *Chicken and Orange Stir-Fry* combines pretty peppers, quick-cooking chicken, and juicy oranges in a subtly sweet chutney-flavored sauce.

HALIBUT WITH GARDEN-STYLE MARINARA SAUCE

At 116 calories per serving, this dynamite fish dish suits dieters, families who want to eat more healthfully, and anyone who wants a full-flavored yet fast meal.

  2 fresh *or* frozen* cod, halibut, salmon, *or* shark steaks, 1 inch thick (about 1 pound total)
1½ cups water
  ½ teaspoon lemon-pepper seasoning
  1 cup thinly sliced zucchini *and/or* yellow summer squash
  ½ of a small onion, sliced and separated into rings
  1 clove garlic, minced
  ¼ cup water
1½ teaspoons snipped fresh oregano *or* ½ teaspoon dried oregano, crushed
  ½ of a 14½-ounce can (1 cup) stewed tomatoes
  2 teaspoons cornstarch
     Dash bottled hot pepper sauce

◆ **Halve** fish. Place the 1½ cups water and *half* of the lemon-pepper seasoning in a large skillet. Bring to boiling; add fish. Return to boiling; reduce heat. Simmer, covered, for 8 to 12 minutes for fresh fish (12 to 18 minutes for frozen fish) or until fish flakes easily with a fork. Transfer fish to a serving platter. Cover to keep warm.

◆ **Meanwhile, for sauce,** combine zucchini, onion, garlic, the ¼ cup water, the oregano, and the remaining lemon-pepper seasoning in a medium saucepan. Bring to boiling; reduce heat. Simmer, covered, about 4 minutes or until vegetables are nearly tender; drain.

◆ **Combine** *undrained* tomatoes, cornstarch, and hot pepper sauce in a small bowl. Stir into vegetables. Cook and stir until thickened and bubbly. Cook and stir for 2 minutes more. To serve, spoon sauce over fish. Makes 4 servings.

◆ ***Note:** Thaw fish, if frozen. To quick-thaw, see tip, *page 19.*

NUTRITION FACTS PER SERVING: 116 calories, 20 g protein, 7 g carbohydrate, 1 g fat, 45 mg cholesterol, 1 g dietary fiber, 346 mg sodium.

SOLE WITH SPINACH AND PLUM TOMATOES

Enjoy this elegant entrée with a clear conscience—it has only 2 grams of fat per serving!

- 1 pound fresh *or* frozen* skinless sole, flounder, *or* whitefish fillets
- 1 10-ounce package frozen chopped spinach, thawed and well drained
- 1 small onion, finely chopped (⅓ cup)
- 2 tablespoons snipped fresh parsley
- 2 cloves garlic, minced
- ½ teaspoon dried oregano, crushed
- ½ teaspoon finely shredded orange peel
- ¼ teaspoon salt
- ¼ teaspoon pepper
- 2 Roma tomatoes

◆ **Set oven** to 400°. Cut fish into serving-size pieces.

◆ **Stir** together spinach, onion, parsley, garlic, oregano, and orange peel in a medium bowl. Place *one-fourth* of the spinach mixture in each of 4 individual casseroles. Place one fish portion in each casserole. Sprinkle with salt and pepper. Cover casseroles with foil. Bake for 5 minutes. Remove foil.

◆ **Meanwhile,** chop tomatoes. Sprinkle tomatoes over casseroles. Bake, uncovered, for 5 to 7 minutes more or until fish flakes easily with a fork. Makes 4 servings.

◆ ***Note:** Thaw fish, if frozen. To quick-thaw, see tip, *page 19.*

NUTRITION FACTS PER SERVING: 139 calories, 24 g protein, 7 g carbohydrate, 2 g fat, 60 mg cholesterol, 2 g dietary fiber, 291 mg sodium.

FAST AND FABULOUS FISH

When you're looking for a fast, healthy meal, there's no need to go out for dinner. You can bake or broil fish in minutes. Add even more flavor to fish dinners with these quick fixes.

• Use your favorite nonfat salad dressing as a dipping sauce.

• Stir together nonfat plain yogurt with chopped, seeded cucumber and a little dillweed for a fresh-tasting topper.

• Or, try this updated version of tartar sauce: Stir together ¼ cup *plain nonfat yogurt,* 2 tablespoons *nonfat mayonnaise dressing,* 2 tablespoons snipped *chutney,* and 1 teaspoon *balsamic vinegar* or *white wine vinegar.* Makes ⅓ cup.

TURKEY AND SHRIMP JAMBALAYA

To cut the fat in this Cajun classic, we've replaced the traditional andouille sausage with smoked turkey sausage.

- 1 14½-ounce can reduced-sodium tomatoes, cut up
- 1 large onion, finely chopped (1 cup)
- ½ cup reduced-sodium chicken broth
- 2 tablespoons tomato paste
- 3 cloves garlic, minced
- 1 bay leaf
- 1 teaspoon dried Italian seasoning, crushed
- ½ teaspoon chili powder
- ¼ teaspoon black pepper
  Few dashes bottled hot pepper sauce
- 2 medium green peppers, chopped (1½ cups)
- 8 ounces frozen peeled, cooked medium shrimp, thawed
- 1 cup quick-cooking rice
- 4 ounces fully cooked smoked turkey sausage, halved lengthwise and cut into ¼-inch-thick slices
  Lemon wedges (optional)

◆ **Combine** *undrained* tomatoes, onion, broth, tomato paste, garlic, bay leaf, Italian seasoning, chili powder, black pepper, and hot pepper sauce in a large saucepan.

◆ **Bring** mixture to boiling; reduce heat. Simmer, covered, for 5 minutes. Stir in green pepper, shrimp, *uncooked* rice, and sausage. Return to boiling; reduce heat. Simmer, covered, about 5 minutes or until mixture is heated through and rice is tender. Stir mixture. Discard bay leaf. Serve with lemon wedges, if desired. Makes 4 servings.

NUTRITION FACTS PER SERVING: 255 calories, 21 g protein, 35 g carbohydrate, 3 g fat, 129 mg cholesterol, 2 g dietary fiber, 486 mg sodium.

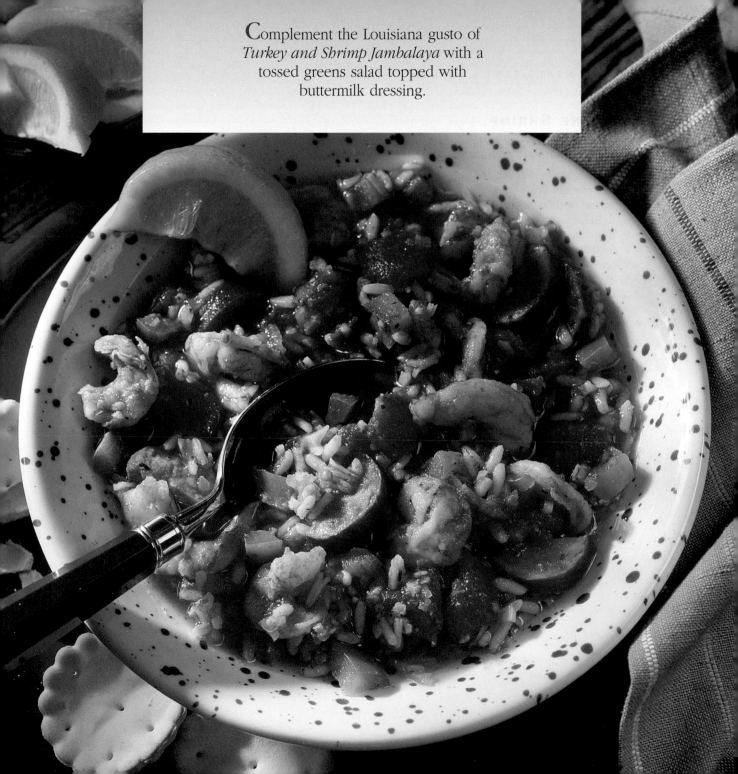

Complement the Louisiana gusto of *Turkey and Shrimp Jambalaya* with a tossed greens salad topped with buttermilk dressing.

SUNSHINE SHRIMP

The peeled and deveined shrimp in this recipe is a real time-saver. If you're planning to peel it yourself, start with 1½ pounds of unpeeled shrimp. Pictured on pages 26–27.

 1 cup couscous *or* quick-cooking rice
 ½ cup chicken broth
 1 pound fresh *or* frozen* peeled and deveined large shrimp
 2 to 2½ teaspoons curry powder
 1 8-ounce carton plain fat-free yogurt
 2 tablespoons all-purpose flour
 ¼ teaspoon ground allspice
 1 8-ounce can sliced bamboo shoots, drained
 3 green onions, bias sliced (⅓ cup)

◆ **Prepare** couscous or rice according to package directions; keep warm.

◆ **Meanwhile,** pour chicken broth into a large skillet; heat to boiling. Add shrimp and curry powder. Cook, uncovered, for 1 to 3 minutes or just until shrimp turn opaque. Remove shrimp with slotted spoon; set aside. Reserve broth in skillet.

◆ **Stir** together yogurt, flour, and allspice in a small bowl. Stir yogurt mixture, bamboo shoots, and green onions into the broth in the skillet. Cook and stir over medium heat until thickened and bubbly. Cook and stir for 1 minute more. Stir in shrimp; heat through. Season to taste with salt and pepper. Spoon over couscous. Makes 4 servings.

◆ ***Note:** Thaw shrimp, if frozen. To quick-thaw, see tip, *page 19.*

NUTRITION FACTS PER SERVING: 320 calories, 30 g protein, 45 g carbohydrate, 2 g fat, 176 mg cholesterol, 8 g dietary fiber, 344 mg sodium.

MANHATTAN CLAM CHOWDER

Tomato-based Manhattan Clam Chowder is usually lower in fat and calories than its milk-based cousin from New England. Our recipe is no exception—check out the nutrition facts below.

2   6½-ounce cans minced clams
    Nonstick spray coating
2   slices turkey bacon, chopped
2   medium potatoes, peeled and finely chopped (2 cups)
1   large onion, chopped (1 cup)
2   stalks celery, chopped (1 cup)
½   teaspoon dried basil *or* marjoram, crushed
¼   teaspoon pepper
2   14½-ounce cans reduced-sodium tomatoes, cut up

◆ **Drain** clams, reserving juice. If necessary, add water to clam juice to equal *1½ cups* liquid. Set aside.

◆ **Spray** an unheated large saucepan with nonstick coating. Preheat over medium heat. Add bacon; cook until lightly browned. Remove bacon from pan; set aside.

◆ **Stir** together the clam juice, potatoes, onion, celery, basil, and pepper in the saucepan. Bring to boiling; reduce heat. Simmer, covered, for 10 to 15 minutes or until the vegetables are tender. Add *undrained* tomatoes; heat through.

◆ **Mash** the vegetables slightly with the back of a fork against the side of the pan. Stir in the clams; heat through. To serve, sprinkle with bacon. Makes 4 servings.

NUTRITION FACTS PER SERVING: 186 calories, 13 g protein, 31 g carbohydrate, 3 g fat, 62 mg cholesterol, 3 g dietary fiber, 210 mg sodium.

PORK MEDAILLONS WITH APPLE-YOGURT SAUCE

Pound the slices of pork tenderloin to a ½-inch thickness so they cook quickly and evenly.

 12 ounces pork tenderloin
      Nonstick spray coating
  1 cup thinly sliced apple
 ½ cup apple juice *or* apple cider
  1 small onion, chopped (⅓ cup)
 ¼ teaspoon salt
 ¼ teaspoon dried sage, crushed
  1 8-ounce carton plain low-fat yogurt
  2 tablespoons all-purpose flour
  2 cups hot cooked spinach fettuccine *or* noodles
      Snipped chives (optional)
      Tiny red onions, halved (optional)
      Fresh sage sprigs (optional)

◆ **Trim** separable fat from pork. Cut pork crosswise into 1-inch-thick slices. Place slices of pork between 2 sheets of plastic wrap. Lightly pound the meat with the flat side of a meat mallet to ½-inch thickness.

◆ **Spray** an unheated 12-inch skillet with nonstick coating. Preheat over medium heat. Add pork slices; cook for 6 to 7 minutes or until no longer pink, turning once. Remove pork from skillet; keep warm.

◆ **For sauce,** add apple slices, apple juice, onion, salt, and sage to skillet. Cook, covered, about 4 minutes or until onion is tender. Remove apple slices and onion with a slotted spoon.

◆ **Meanwhile,** stir together yogurt and flour. Add yogurt mixture to skillet. Cook and stir until thickened and bubbly. Cook and stir for 1 minute more. Arrange pork, fettuccine, apple slices, and onion on 4 individual serving plates. Spoon some of the sauce over each serving. Sprinkle with snipped chives and garnish with red onion halves and sage sprigs, if desired. Pass remaining sauce. Makes 4 servings.

NUTRITION FACTS PER SERVING: 288 calories, 19 g protein, 36 g carbohydrate, 7 g fat, 42 mg cholesterol, 2 g dietary fiber, 204 mg sodium.

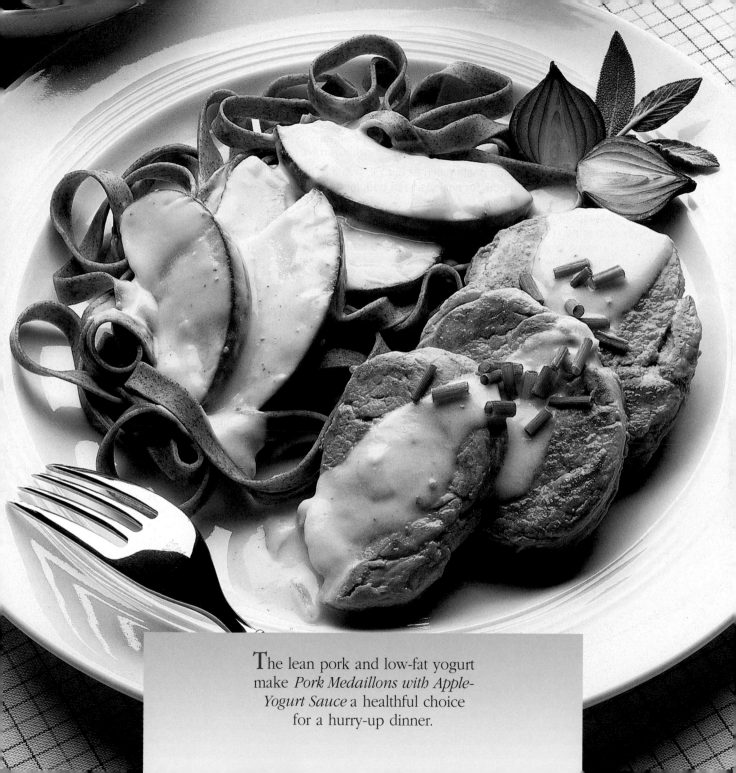

The lean pork and low-fat yogurt make *Pork Medaillons with Apple-Yogurt Sauce* a healthful choice for a hurry-up dinner.

PICATTA-STYLE PORK

Create a no-fat picatta sauce from lemon juice and an envelope of butter-flavored sprinkles,
which can be found in the spice section of your supermarket.

    6 ounces packaged dried pasta (such as cut ziti, linguine, *or* angel hair)
   12 ounces thinly sliced pork for scaloppine *or* pork tenderloin
       Nonstick spray coating
    2 tablespoons beef *or* chicken broth
   ¼ cup lemon juice
    1 ½-ounce envelope butter-flavored sprinkles (8 teaspoons)
    1 teaspoon Dijon-style mustard
   ⅛ teaspoon pepper

◆ **Cook** pasta according to package directions. Drain and keep warm.

◆ **Meanwhile,** set oven to broil. If using pork tenderloin, slice meat ½ inch thick. Place
tenderloin slices between 2 sheets of plastic wrap. Lightly pound with flat side of meat mallet
to ⅛-inch thickness.

◆ **Spray** the unheated rack of a broiler pan generously with nonstick coating. Arrange pork
scaloppine or pounded pork tenderloin slices on rack of broiler pan; brush generously with
broth. Broil for 4 to 6 minutes or until no longer pink, turning and brushing with broth once.

◆ **Meanwhile,** for sauce, stir together lemon juice, butter-flavored sprinkles, mustard, and
pepper in a small saucepan. Heat through over low heat.

◆ **To serve,** pour *half* of the sauce over hot pasta; toss to coat. Arrange pasta and pork on
4 individual serving plates. Spoon remaining sauce over meat. Makes 4 servings.

NUTRITION FACTS PER SERVING: 288 calories, 24 g protein, 38 g carbohydrate, 4 g fat, 59 mg cholesterol, 0 g dietary fiber, 241 mg sodium.

WINE-SAUCED PORK MEDAILLONS

12 ounces pork tenderloin
   Nonstick spray coating
 4 shallots *or* 1 small onion, thinly sliced
½ cup dry white wine
 2 tablespoons red currant jelly
 2 teaspoons Dijon-style mustard

◆ **Trim** separable fat from pork. Cut pork crosswise into 1-inch-thick slices. Place slices of pork between 2 sheets of plastic wrap. Lightly pound with flat side of meat mallet to ¼-inch thickness.

◆ **Spray** an unheated nonstick large skillet with nonstick coating. Preheat over medium heat. Add *half* of the pork; cook for 3 to 4 minutes or until no longer pink, turning once. Remove from skillet; keep warm. Repeat with remaining pork.

◆ **Add** shallots to skillet; cook for 1 minute. Stir in wine, jelly, and mustard. Bring to boiling; cook and stir about 2 minutes or until slightly thickened. Serve over pork. Serves 4.

NUTRITION FACTS PER SERVING: 164 calories, 19 g protein, 9 g carbohydrate, 4 g fat, 60 mg cholesterol, 0 g dietary fiber, 111 mg sodium.

COOKING WITH NONSTICK SPRAY COATING

Reducing the fat in your diet can be as simple as substituting nonstick spray coating for the oil, shortening, or butter you would normally use in your baking pans and skillets. Nonstick spray coatings are available in several flavors—butter, olive oil, as well as unflavored—so you can choose the one that best fits the food you're cooking.

How do these sprays work? Vegetable oil and lecithin (from soybeans) prevent sticking; a small amount of alcohol is added to some sprays for clarity. A 1-second spray covers a 10-inch skillet, and contains less than 1 gram of fat and 7 calories. Try these techniques when spraying.

• Spray sparingly. The longer you spray, the more oil—and calories—you'll add to your food.

• Spray only onto unheated pans, skillets, or other utensils; the coating can burn or smoke if applied to hot surfaces.

• Use medium heat when cooking in a utensil sprayed with nonstick coating. High heat causes the coating to smoke.

BLACKENED BEEF STIR-FRY

Steak is great—as long as you don't overindulge. Here, strips of beef sirloin steak are extended with a bounty of vegetables.

12 ounces boneless beef sirloin steak *or* top round steak*, cut ½ to ¾ inch thick
 1 teaspoon paprika
 ½ teaspoon garlic powder
 ¼ teaspoon dried thyme, crushed
 ¼ teaspoon black pepper
 ⅛ teaspoon salt
 ⅛ to ¼ teaspoon ground red pepper
 ⅔ cup beef broth
 2 tablespoons tomato paste
 2 teaspoons cornstarch
   Nonstick spray coating
 2 cups broccoli flowerets
 1 medium carrot, bias sliced (½ cup)
 2 cups sliced fresh mushrooms
 ½ cup bias-sliced green onions
 1 8-ounce package frozen baby corn, thawed
 2 tablespoons beef broth
 2 cups hot cooked rice

◆ **Trim** separable fat from beef. Thinly slice beef across the grain into bite-size strips. Stir together paprika, garlic powder, thyme, black pepper, salt, and red pepper in a medium bowl. Add beef strips; toss to coat well.

◆ **For sauce,** stir together the ⅔ cup beef broth, the tomato paste, and cornstarch in a small bowl; set aside.

◆ **Spray** an unheated wok or 12-inch skillet with nonstick coating. Preheat over medium heat. Add broccoli and carrot; stir-fry for 3 minutes. Add mushrooms and green onions; stir-fry 2 minutes more. Add corn; stir-fry 2 minutes more. Remove from wok. Carefully add the 2 tablespoons broth to wok. Add the meat; stir-fry for 2 to 3 minutes or until desired doneness.

◆ **Push** meat from center of wok. Stir sauce; pour into center of wok. Cook and stir until thickened and bubbly. Return vegetables to wok. Stir to coat all ingredients with sauce. Cook and stir about 1 minute more or until heated through. Serve over hot cooked rice. Makes 4 servings.

◆ ***Note:** Partially freeze the beef to make it easier to slice.

NUTRITION FACTS PER SERVING: 303 calories, 24 g protein, 41 g carbohydrate, 5 g fat, 49 mg cholesterol, 5 g dietary fiber, 351 mg sodium.

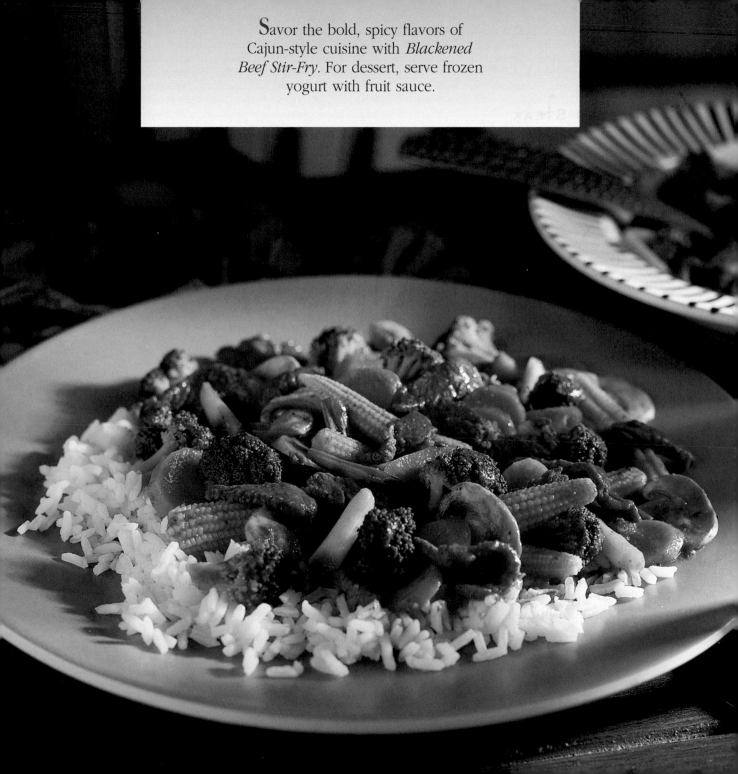

Savor the bold, spicy flavors of Cajun-style cuisine with *Blackened Beef Stir-Fry*. For dessert, serve frozen yogurt with fruit sauce.

PEPPER STEAK

Busy and health-conscious cooks love to stir-fry. They can cook food using a minimum of fat, in a minimum amount of time.

12	ounces boneless beef sirloin steak*, cut ½ to ¾ inch thick
½	cup water
2	tablespoons light soy sauce *or* 1 tablespoon Worcestershire sauce
1	tablespoon cornstarch
½	teaspoon instant beef bouillon granules
	Dash pepper
6	ounces packaged dried fettuccine
	Nonstick spray coating
1	medium onion, cut into thin wedges
1	clove garlic, minced
1	medium green pepper, cut into 1-inch pieces
1	tablespoon cooking oil
2	medium tomatoes, cut into thin wedges

◆ **Trim** separable fat from beef. Thinly slice beef across the grain into bite-size strips.

◆ **For sauce,** stir together the water, soy sauce, cornstarch, bouillon granules, and pepper in a small mixing bowl; set aside.

◆ **Cook** the fettuccine according to the package directions, *except* omit the cooking oil and salt; drain. Keep warm.

◆ **Meanwhile,** spray an unheated wok or large skillet with nonstick coating. Preheat over medium heat. Add the onion and garlic; stir-fry for 1 minute. Add the green pepper; stir-fry about 2 minutes more or until vegetables are crisp-tender. Remove vegetables from the wok.

◆ **Pour** oil into hot wok. Add the beef; stir-fry for 2 to 3 minutes or until desired doneness. Push beef from the center of the wok. Stir the sauce; pour into center of wok. Cook and stir until thickened and bubbly.

◆ **Return** the cooked vegetables to the wok. Stir to coat all ingredients with sauce. Cook and stir about 1 minute more or until heated through. Gently stir in the tomato wedges; heat through. Serve over hot cooked fettuccine. Makes 4 servings.

◆ ***Note:** Partially freeze the beef to make it easier to slice.

NUTRITION FACTS PER SERVING: 397 calories, 31 g protein, 41 g carbohydrate, 11 g fat, 69 mg cholesterol, 2 g dietary fiber, 446 mg sodium.

Sloppy Joes

Oat bran stirred into the sandwich mixture thickens the sauce, and boosts the fiber content of the recipe.

- 8 ounces 90% lean ground beef
- 1 large onion, chopped (1 cup)
- 1 medium green pepper, chopped (¾ cup)
- 1 clove garlic, minced
- ½ of a 14½-ounce can reduced-sodium tomatoes, cut up
- ¼ cup water
- 2 tablespoons oat bran
- 1 tablespoon vinegar
- 2 teaspoons brown sugar
- 1 to 1½ teaspoons chili powder
- 1 teaspoon Worcestershire sauce
- ⅛ teaspoon salt
  Dash bottled hot pepper sauce
- 5 hamburger buns, split and toasted

◆ **Cook** and stir ground beef, onion, green pepper, and garlic in a large skillet over medium-high heat until beef is brown. Drain fat.

◆ **Stir in** *undrained* tomatoes, the water, oat bran, vinegar, brown sugar, chili powder, Worcestershire sauce, salt, and hot pepper sauce. Bring to boiling; reduce heat. Simmer, covered, for 5 minutes. If necessary, uncover and simmer for 3 to 5 minutes more or until mixture is desired consistency. Spoon mixture onto hamburger buns. Makes 5 servings.

NUTRITION FACTS PER SERVING: 225 calories, 13 g protein, 29 g carbohydrate, 7 g fat, 29 mg cholesterol, 2 g dietary fiber, 335 mg sodium.

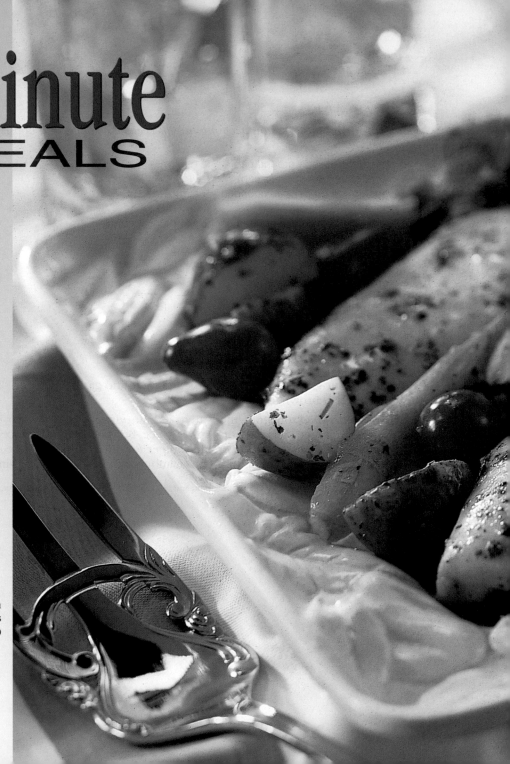

30-Minute MEALS

Think quick! And think healthy! Give your kitchen just 30 minutes, and you'll get a memorable meal to linger over with friends and family. Featuring the fresh taste of good-for-you ingredients, these recipes show that healthful meals can be special meals, too.

Roasted Italian Chicken and Vegetables (see recipe, *page 63*)

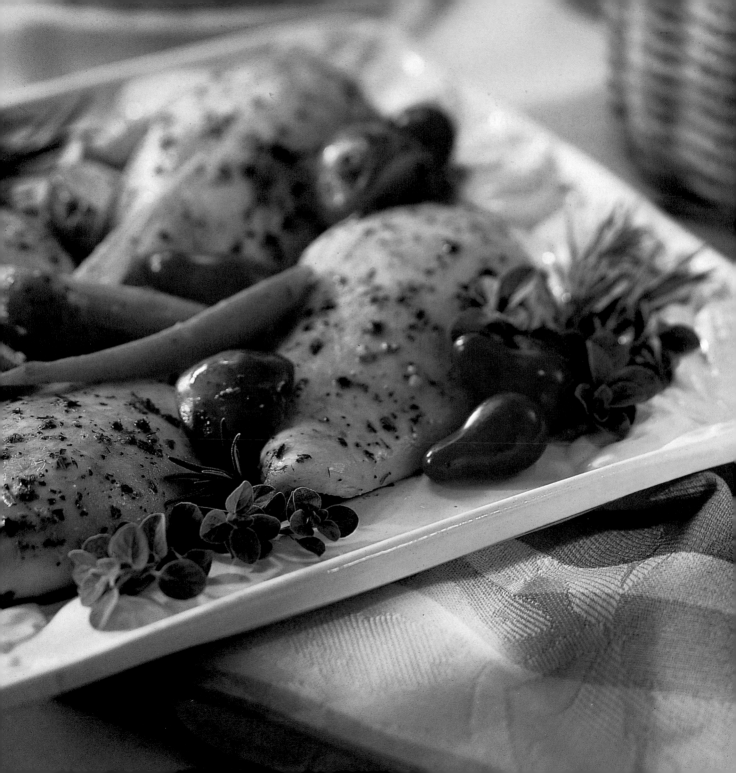

CHICKEN CACCIATORE

Opt for chicken breasts instead of thighs to trim even more fat from this one-dish meal.

  8 skinless, boneless chicken thighs (1¼ pounds total) *or* 4 medium skinless, boneless chicken
        breast halves (1 pound total)
       Nonstick spray coating
  1 14½-ounce can reduced-sodium stewed tomatoes
  1 cup purchased spaghetti sauce
  1 2½-ounce jar sliced mushrooms, drained (optional)
  6 ounces packaged dried linguine *or* fettuccine
  1 tablespoon cornstarch
  1 tablespoon cold water
  2 cups frozen pepper stir-fry vegetables (yellow, green, and red sweet peppers and onions)
  ½ cup shredded reduced-fat mozzarella cheese (optional)

◆ **Rinse** chicken; pat dry with paper towels. Spray an unheated large skillet with nonstick coating. Preheat over medium heat. Add chicken; cook for 5 minutes, turning once. Add *undrained* stewed tomatoes, spaghetti sauce, and, if desired, mushrooms. Bring to boiling; reduce heat. Simmer, covered, about 15 minutes or until chicken is tender and no longer pink.

◆ **Meanwhile,** cook linguine according to package directions, *except* omit the oil and salt; drain. Keep warm.

◆ **Combine** cornstarch and cold water in a small bowl; add to skillet. Cook and stir until thickened and bubbly. Stir in stir-fry vegetables. Cook and stir for 2 minutes more. Serve over hot cooked pasta. Sprinkle with cheese, if desired. Makes 4 servings.

NUTRITION FACTS PER SERVING: 359 calories, 16 g protein, 57 g carbohydrate, 7 g fat, 27 mg cholesterol, 3 g dietary fiber, 390 mg sodium.

ROASTED ITALIAN CHICKEN AND VEGETABLES

Fresh oregano and rosemary sprigs may be used to embellish this easy oven meal, pictured on pages 60–61.

    16 baby carrots, halved lengthwise
    12 tiny new potatoes, halved
    ⅓ cup fat-free Italian salad dressing
     1 teaspoon dried Italian seasoning, crushed
     4 small skinless, boneless chicken breast halves (12 ounces total)
        Nonstick spray coating
    12 yellow *or* red pear-shaped *or* cherry tomatoes

◆ **Set oven** to 375°. Add a small amount of water to a 2-quart saucepan; bring to boiling. Add carrots and potatoes; return to boiling. Cook, covered, for 8 minutes.

◆ **Meanwhile,** stir together salad dressing, Italian seasoning, and ⅛ teaspoon *pepper* in a bowl. Rinse chicken; pat dry with paper towels. Spray a 9x9x2-inch baking pan with nonstick coating. Brush chicken with *half* of the dressing mixture. Place chicken in baking pan. Bake, uncovered, for 10 minutes.

◆ **Drain** vegetables and toss with remaining salad dressing mixture. Pour over chicken. Return to oven and bake about 5 minutes more or until chicken is tender and no longer pink.

◆ **Transfer** chicken to a serving platter. Toss tomatoes with vegetables. Arrange vegetables around chicken; brush chicken and vegetables with pan drippings. Makes 4 servings.

NUTRITION FACTS PER SERVING: 254 calories, 20 g protein, 37 g carbohydrate, 3 g fat, 45 mg cholesterol, 5 g dietary fiber, 384 mg sodium.

MICROWAVE QUICK-THAW FOR POULTRY

When you're in a hurry, use your microwave oven to thaw poultry. Unwrap poultry and place it on a microwave-safe dish. Cover; defrost on 30 percent power (medium-low) for time listed *below*. Turn or separate poultry halfway through defrosting time. Let stand a few minutes to complete thawing.

- Chicken, cut up (2½ to 3 pounds): 15 to 17 minutes
- Chicken breasts, boneless, skinless (1½ pounds): 12 to 14 minutes
- Chicken or turkey, ground (1 pound): 10 to 12 minutes
- Turkey breast tenderloin steaks (1 pound): 8 to 10 minutes

MANGO CHICKEN

To cut a mango, slice through the fruit, sliding a sharp knife next to the seed. Repeat on the other side of the seed. Then cut away all the meat that remains around the seed. Peel all pieces.

12 ounces skinless, boneless chicken breast halves *or* thighs
½ cup reduced-sodium chicken broth
 2 teaspoons finely shredded lime peel *or* orange peel
 2 tablespoons lime juice
 2 teaspoons brown sugar
 2 teaspoons curry powder
 1 teaspoon cornstarch
    Nonstick spray coating
 1 large red onion, sliced (1 cup)
 2 cloves garlic, minced
 2 teaspoons peanut oil *or* cooking oil
 2 cups chopped, peeled mango *or* papaya
 2 cups hot cooked rice
    Lime peel, cut into fine strips (optional)

◆ **Rinse** chicken; pat dry with paper towels. Cut chicken into bite-size strips; set aside.

◆ **For sauce,** stir together broth, the shredded lime peel, lime juice, brown sugar, curry powder, and cornstarch in a small bowl; set aside.

◆ **Spray** an unheated large wok or 12-inch skillet with nonstick coating. Preheat over medium heat. Add onion and garlic; stir-fry about 3 minutes or until crisp-tender. Remove from wok.

◆ **Pour** oil into hot wok. Add the chicken; stir-fry for 2 to 3 minutes or until chicken is tender and no longer pink.

◆ **Push** chicken from center of wok. Stir sauce; pour into center of wok. Cook and stir until thickened and bubbly. Return onion mixture to the wok. Add mango. Stir to coat all ingredients with sauce. Cook and stir about 2 minutes more or until heated through. Serve over hot cooked rice. Garnish with the strips of lime peel, if desired. Makes 4 servings.

NUTRITION FACTS PER SERVING: 287 calories, 20 g protein, 40 g carbohydrate, 5 g fat, 45 mg cholesterol, 2 g dietary fiber, 125 mg sodium.

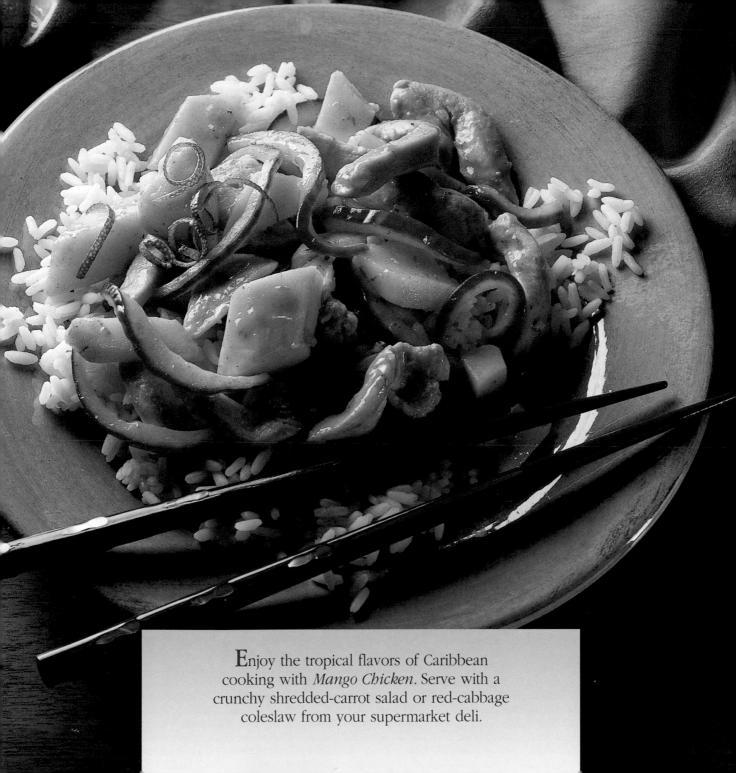

Enjoy the tropical flavors of Caribbean cooking with *Mango Chicken*. Serve with a crunchy shredded-carrot salad or red-cabbage coleslaw from your supermarket deli.

CHICKEN AND RASPBERRY SPINACH SALAD

Vary the fruit in this salad with the season. Try strawberries if you can't find fresh raspberries; use cantaloupe or oranges when papaya, nectarines, or peaches aren't available.

- 4 medium skinless, boneless chicken breast halves (1 pound total)
- ¼ cup raspberry vinegar *or* white wine vinegar
- 2 tablespoons salad oil
- 1 tablespoon honey
- ½ teaspoon finely shredded orange peel
- ¼ teaspoon salt
- ¼ teaspoon pepper
- ⅓ cup water
- ¼ cup orange juice
- 8 to 10 cups purchased torn fresh spinach *or* mixed greens
- 1 cup fresh raspberries
- 2 papayas, peeled, seeded, and cut into thin slices, *or* 4 medium nectarines *or* peaches, pitted and cut into thin slices

◆ **Rinse** chicken; pat dry with paper towels. Set aside.

◆ **For dressing,** combine vinegar, salad oil, honey, orange peel, salt, and pepper in a small screw-top jar. Cover and shake well. Chill dressing until needed.

◆ **Combine** the water and orange juice in a medium skillet. Bring to boiling; add chicken. Return to boiling; reduce heat. Simmer, covered, for 12 to 15 minutes or until chicken is tender and no longer pink. Remove chicken from skillet; cool slightly. Cut chicken into bite-size pieces.

◆ **Combine** warm chicken and spinach in a large bowl. Shake dressing; add dressing and raspberries to spinach mixture. Toss gently. Divide salad mixture among 4 individual serving plates. Top each salad with several papaya slices, arranging them in a fan. Serve immediately. Makes 4 main-dish servings.

NUTRITION FACTS PER SERVING: 334 calories, 21 g protein, 42 g carbohydrate, 10 g fat, 45 mg cholesterol, 9 g dietary fiber, 278 mg sodium.

BAKED SOLE AND CORN SALSA

1 pound fresh *or* frozen* fish fillets (such as sole, flounder, *or* haddock), ½ inch thick
Nonstick spray coating
1½ cups salsa
½ cup frozen whole kernel corn

◆ **Set oven** to 375°. Cut fish into serving-size portions. Spray a 2-quart rectangular baking dish with nonstick coating. Place fish in baking dish, turning under any thin edges.

◆ **Combine** salsa and corn in a small mixing bowl. Spoon over fish. Bake, uncovered, for 20 to 25 minutes or until fish flakes easily with a fork. Transfer fish and salsa topping to individual serving plates using a slotted spoon. Makes 4 servings.

◆ ***Note:** To quick-thaw fish, see tip, *page 19.*

NUTRITION FACTS PER SERVING: 130 calories, 20 g protein, 9 g carbohydrate, 3 g fat, 45 mg cholesterol, 0 g dietary fiber, 398 mg sodium.

VINEGAR MAKES A SPLASH

Supermarket shelves are brimming with varieties of vinegars, from spirited and fruity to aged and aromatic. Here's a rundown of new and traditional vinegar choices:

• Cider vinegar is made from fermented apples, which add a tawny color and slight fruity flavor.

• White or distilled vinegar is made from grains such as corn, rye, and barley. Its very tart flavor lends itself to pickling.

• Malt vinegar, made from ale and fermented potatoes or grain, is brownish in color and yeasty in flavor. It's best known as an accompaniment to English fish and chips, but can be used for recipes calling for cider vinegar.

• Wine vinegars are made from wine, sherry, or champagne, and are the mildest and most versatile of all vinegars.

• Rice wine vinegar starts with sake and has a clean, mild, and slightly sweet taste.

• Fruit and herb vinegars are made from either cider, white, or wine vinegars, and flavored with the natural flavors of fruits and herbs.

• Balsamic vinegar is made from the unfermented juice of high-sugar grapes and is aged in wooden barrels. The finished vinegar is dark brown, and offers a full-bodied flavor.

FLOUNDER DIJON

When time is short, substitute shredded carrot for the julienne strips in the creamy, mustard-flavored vegetable sauce. Shredded carrot cooks much faster than julienne strips.

    4   fresh or frozen* flounder, sole, *or* pompano fillets (12 ounces total)
        Nonstick spray coating
    ½   cup sliced fresh mushrooms
    ⅓   cup sliced zucchini
    ¼   cup carrot cut into thin 1-inch strips
    2   green onions, sliced (¼ cup)
    ¾   cup skim milk
    1½ teaspoons cornstarch
    1½ teaspoons Dijon-style mustard
    1   teaspoon instant chicken bouillon granules

◆ **Set oven** to 450°. Measure thickness of fish. Spray a 2-quart rectangular baking dish with nonstick coating. Place fish in baking dish, turning under any thin edges. Bake until fish flakes easily with a fork. (Allow 4 to 6 minutes for each ½-inch thickness of fish.)

◆ **Meanwhile,** for sauce, spray an unheated medium saucepan with nonstick coating. Preheat saucepan over medium heat. Add mushrooms, zucchini, carrot, and green onions; cook and stir for 3 to 4 minutes or until crisp-tender. Stir together milk, cornstarch, mustard, and bouillon granules. Add milk mixture to vegetables in saucepan. Cook and stir until thickened and bubbly. Cook and stir for 2 minutes more.

◆ **Transfer** fish to individual serving plates. Spoon sauce over fish. Makes 4 servings.

◆ ***Note:** Thaw fish, if frozen. To quick-thaw, see tip, *page 19*.

NUTRITION FACTS PER SERVING: 107 calories, 18 g protein, 5 g carbohydrate, 2 g fat, 46 mg cholesterol, 0 g dietary fiber, 357 mg sodium.

TURKEY APRICOT STIR-FRY

To speed the preparation of this fruit-studded stir-fry, chop the ingredients the night before.

12   ounces turkey breast tenderloin steaks
½   cup apricot *or* peach nectar
3   tablespoons light soy sauce
2   tablespoons rice vinegar *or* white vinegar
1   tablespoon cornstarch
¼   teaspoon ground red pepper
½   cup dried apricot halves, cut in half
      Nonstick spray coating
1   small red sweet pepper, cut into 1-inch pieces
1   small onion, chopped (⅓ cup)
1   tablespoon cooking oil
1   6-ounce package frozen pea pods
2   cups hot cooked couscous *or* rice

◆ **Rinse** turkey; pat dry with paper towels. Thinly slice turkey into bite-size strips. Set aside.

◆ **For sauce,** stir together nectar, soy sauce, vinegar, cornstarch, and ground red pepper in a small bowl. Add apricots. Set aside.

◆ **Spray** an unheated wok or large skillet with nonstick coating. Preheat over medium heat. Add sweet pepper and onion; stir-fry for 2 to 3 minutes or until crisp-tender. Remove vegetables from wok.

◆ **Pour** oil into hot wok. Add the turkey; stir-fry for 2 to 3 minutes or until turkey is tender and no longer pink.

◆ **Push** turkey from center of wok. Stir sauce; pour into center of the wok. Cook and stir until thickened and bubbly. Return cooked vegetables to wok. Add pea pods. Stir to coat all ingredients with sauce. Cook and stir about 1 minute more or until pea pods are heated through. Serve over hot cooked couscous. Makes 4 servings.

NUTRITION FACTS PER SERVING: 317 calories, 23 g protein, 44 g carbohydrate, 6 g fat, 37 mg cholesterol, 7 g dietary fiber, 440 mg sodium.

ROASTED RED SNAPPER

An extra-hot oven cooks the fish quickly—with no turning required.

1 pound fresh *or* frozen* red snapper fillets, 1 inch thick
1 14½-ounce can reduced-sodium tomatoes, cut up
8 green onions, sliced (1 cup)
¼ cup thinly sliced celery
2 tablespoons lemon juice
1 teaspoon dried oregano, crushed
   Nonstick spray coating
¼ teaspoon pepper
¼ teaspoon ground coriander
¼ cup crumbled feta cheese (1 ounce)
2 tablespoons sliced pitted ripe olives
   Parsley sprigs (optional)

◆ **Set oven** to 450°. Cut fish into 4 serving-size portions.

◆ **Combine** *undrained* tomatoes, green onions, celery, lemon juice, and oregano in a large skillet. Bring to boiling; reduce heat. Simmer, uncovered, about 15 minutes or until most of the liquid has evaporated.

◆ **Meanwhile,** spray a 2-quart rectangular baking dish with nonstick coating. Place fish in baking dish, turning under any thin edges. Sprinkle with the pepper and coriander. Bake for 8 to 10 minutes or until fish flakes easily with a fork.

◆ **Transfer** fish to individual serving plates. Spoon sauce over fish. Sprinkle feta cheese and olives over fish. Garnish with parsley sprigs, if desired. Makes 4 servings.

◆ ***Note:** Thaw fish, if frozen. To quick-thaw, see tip, *page 19*.

NUTRITION FACTS PER SERVING: 169 calories, 26 g protein, 7 g carbohydrate, 4 g fat, 48 mg cholesterol, 1 g dietary fiber, 189 mg sodium.

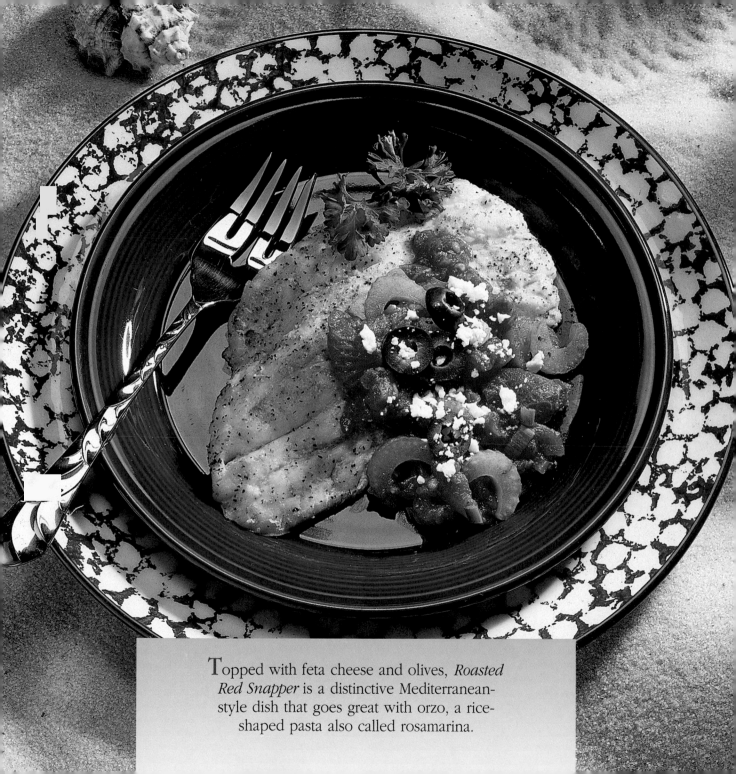

Topped with feta cheese and olives, *Roasted Red Snapper* is a distinctive Mediterranean-style dish that goes great with orzo, a rice-shaped pasta also called rosamarina.

VEGETARIAN CHILI WITH BISCUITS

Your family won't miss the meat in this full-flavored dish. To save time, the dumpling-like biscuits cook in the simmering chili.

- 3 14½-ounce cans reduced-sodium whole tomatoes, cut up
- 1 15-ounce can reduced-sodium garbanzo beans, rinsed and drained
- 1 15-ounce can reduced-sodium kidney beans, rinsed and drained
- 2 stalks celery, chopped (1 cup)
- 1 large onion, chopped (1 cup)
- ½ cup apple juice *or* apple cider
- ½ cup vegetable broth
- 2 teaspoons chili powder
- 1 teaspoon bottled minced garlic
- ½ teaspoon dried oregano, crushed
- ¼ teaspoon pepper
  Sour Cream Biscuits (see recipe, *below*)
- ¾ cup shredded cheddar cheese (3 ounces)

◆ **Stir together** *undrained* tomatoes, garbanzo beans, kidney beans, celery, onion, apple juice, vegetable broth, chili powder, garlic, oregano, and pepper in a 4-quart Dutch oven or kettle. Bring to boiling; reduce heat.

◆ **Drop** Sour Cream Biscuit dough in 8 mounds onto simmering mixture. Cook, covered, about 12 minutes or until a toothpick inserted into biscuits comes out clean. Ladle soup into 8 soup bowls. Place a biscuit on top of each serving and sprinkle with cheese. Makes 8 servings.

◆ **Sour Cream Biscuits:** Stir together ½ cup *all-purpose flour,* ½ cup *whole wheat flour,* 1½ teaspoons *baking powder,* and ⅛ teaspoon *salt* in a medium bowl. Add ½ cup *skim milk* and ¼ cup *light dairy sour cream,* stirring just until mixture is moistened.

NUTRITION FACTS PER SERVING: 257 calories, 15 g protein, 44 g carbohydrate, 6 g fat, 14 mg cholesterol, 8 g dietary fiber, 435 mg sodium.

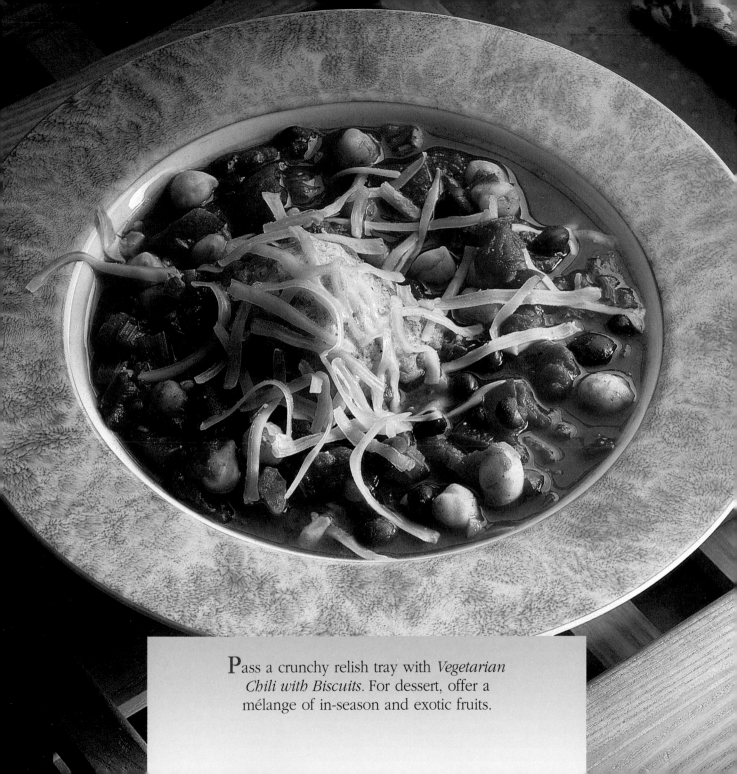

Pass a crunchy relish tray with *Vegetarian Chili with Biscuits*. For dessert, offer a mélange of in-season and exotic fruits.

CURRIED BROCCOLI AND PASTA

Rotini is corkscrew-shaped pasta. Cook the pasta just until it is al dente, which means it is tender, but still firm to the bite.

    8 ounces packaged dried rotini
    3 cups broccoli flowerets
    1 small red *or* green sweet pepper, chopped (½ cup)
    1 8-ounce carton plain fat-free yogurt
    2 tablespoons all-purpose flour
    ⅛ teaspoon salt
    ⅔ cup reduced-sodium chicken broth
    2 teaspoons margarine
    2 teaspoons curry powder
    ½ teaspoon ground cumin
    ¼ cup chopped unsalted peanuts

◆ **Cook** pasta according to package directions, *except* omit salt and add the broccoli and sweet pepper during the last 3 to 4 minutes of cooking; drain.

◆ **Meanwhile,** stir together the yogurt, flour, and salt in a small bowl. Stir in broth and set aside. Place margarine in a large skillet. Heat over medium heat until melted. Stir in curry powder and cumin. Cook and stir for 1 minute. Stir in the yogurt mixture. Cook and stir until thickened and bubbly; cook and stir for 2 minutes more.

◆ **Add** drained pasta mixture to mixture in skillet, tossing to coat pasta. Heat through. Turn into a serving dish. Sprinkle with peanuts. Makes 4 servings.

NUTRITION FACTS PER SERVING: 373 calories, 17 g protein, 60 g carbohydrate, 8 g fat, 1 mg cholesterol, 5 g dietary fiber, 268 mg sodium.

BLACK BEANS AND RICE

1½ cups quick-cooking brown rice
    Nonstick spray coating
  1 large onion, chopped (1 cup)
  1 stalk celery, chopped (½ cup)
  1 medium carrot, thinly sliced (½ cup)
1½ teaspoons bottled minced garlic
  1 15-ounce can reduced-sodium black beans, rinsed and drained
  1 14½-ounce can reduced-sodium stewed tomatoes
 ½ teaspoon ground cumin
 ½ teaspoon dried oregano, crushed
 ¼ teaspoon ground red pepper
  1 green onion, thinly sliced (2 tablespoons) (optional)

◆ **Cook** rice according to package directions, *except* use ¼ teaspoon *salt*. Meanwhile, spray an unheated large saucepan with nonstick coating. Add onion, celery, carrot, and garlic; cook and stir for 4 to 5 minutes. Carefully add drained beans, *undrained* stewed tomatoes, cumin, oregano, red pepper, and ¼ teaspoon *salt*. Bring to boiling; reduce heat. Simmer, uncovered, for 5 to 10 minutes or until desired consistency.

◆ **Serve** bean mixture over rice. Sprinkle with green onion, if desired. Makes 4 servings.

NUTRITION FACTS PER SERVING: 229 calories, 9 g protein, 48 g carbohydrate, 1 g fat, 0 mg cholesterol, 8 g dietary fiber, 454 mg sodium.

MAKE IT MEATLESS

Meatless main dishes are a great way to add variety and good nutrition to your family's meals. Good, low-fat, nonmeat sources of protein include beans, lentils, split peas, tofu, low-fat dairy products, and refrigerated or frozen egg products.

True vegetarians must plan their meatless meals a little more carefully than occasional vegetarians do. That's because plant proteins are not as high in quality as animal proteins. By combining legumes (like beans and lentils) with grains, nuts, seeds, milk, or egg products, vegetarians can mimic the high-quality proteins found in animal products.

Dairy products contain complete proteins, but also may contain more fat and calories than you want, unless you make smart, low-fat dairy choices. Refrigerated and frozen egg substitutes contain the same protein as whole eggs, with less fat and no cholesterol.

THAI BEEF SALAD

Thai cooking is characteristically spicy, and this salad, flavored with basil, mint, ginger, garlic, and jalapeños, is no exception.

   1 large yellow, red, *or* green sweet pepper, cut into bite-size strips
   ½ of a medium cucumber, cut into bite-size strips
   ¼ cup lime juice
   2 tablespoons brown sugar
   2 tablespoons light soy sauce
   1 teaspoon dried basil, crushed
   ½ teaspoon dried mint, crushed
   ¼ teaspoon ground ginger
   8 ounces beef sirloin steak*
      Nonstick spray coating
   1 clove garlic, minced
   1 jalapeño pepper, seeded and minced**
   5 cups purchased torn mixed salad greens
      Lime wedges (optional)

◆ **Combine** sweet pepper and cucumber in a medium bowl.

◆ **For dressing,** stir together lime juice, brown sugar, soy sauce, basil, mint, and ginger in a small bowl. Set aside.

◆ **Trim** separable fat from beef. Thinly slice beef across the grain into bite-size strips. Spray an unheated large skillet with nonstick coating. Preheat over medium heat. Add beef, garlic, and jalapeño pepper; stir-fry for 3 to 4 minutes or until beef is desired doneness. Remove beef mixture from skillet. Add to vegetable mixture. Toss gently.

◆ **Add** dressing to skillet. Bring to boiling. Remove from heat.

◆ **Divide** greens among 4 individual serving plates. Spoon beef-vegetable mixture over the greens. Drizzle dressing over all. Serve with lime wedges, if desired. Serve immediately. Makes 4 servings.

◆ ***Note:** Partially freeze the beef to make it easier to slice.

◆ ****Note:** Protect your hands when working with hot peppers by wearing plastic or rubber gloves or working with plastic bags on your hands. If your bare hands touch the peppers, wash your hands and under your nails thoroughly with soap and water. Avoid rubbing your mouth, nose, eyes, or ears when working with hot peppers.

NUTRITION FACTS PER SERVING: 160 calories, 15 g protein, 13 g carbohydrate, 6 g fat, 38 mg cholesterol, 1 g dietary fiber, 313 mg sodium.

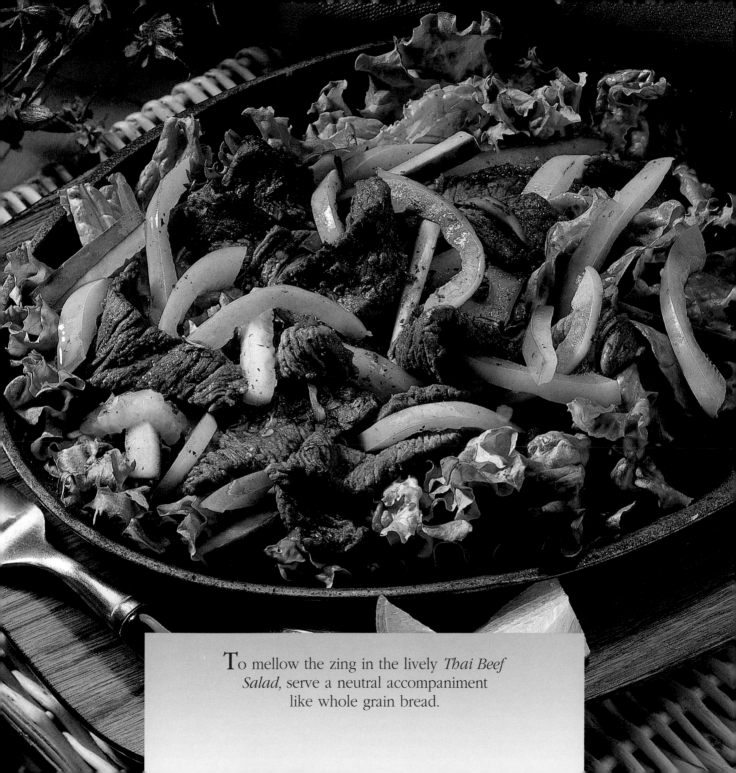

To mellow the zing in the lively *Thai Beef Salad,* serve a neutral accompaniment like whole grain bread.

CHILI-MAC SKILLET

An old favorite takes a new turn, thanks to lean ground beef, reduced-fat cheese, and low-sodium tomatoes and beans. Check the label on the ground beef to make sure it is at least 90 percent lean (10 percent fat). Drain well after browning.

8   ounces 90% lean ground beef
1   medium onion, chopped (½ cup)
1   15½-ounce can light-sodium red kidney beans, rinsed and drained
1   8-ounce can low-sodium tomato sauce
½   of a 14½-ounce can (1 cup) low-sodium tomatoes, cut up
½   cup packaged dried elbow macaroni
1   small green pepper, chopped (½ cup)
¼   cup water
1   tablespoon chili powder
½   teaspoon garlic salt
¼   cup shredded reduced-fat Monterey Jack cheese *or* cheddar cheese (1 ounce)

◆ **Cook** and stir the ground beef and onion in a large skillet over medium-high heat until beef is brown. Drain fat. Stir in the kidney beans, tomato sauce, *undrained* tomatoes, *uncooked* macaroni, green pepper, water, chili powder, and garlic salt. Bring to boiling; reduce heat. Simmer, covered, for 20 minutes, stirring often.

◆ **Remove** skillet from heat. Sprinkle meat mixture with cheese. Cover and let stand about 2 minutes or until the cheese melts. Makes 4 servings.

NUTRITION FACTS PER SERVING: 313 calories, 22 g protein, 40 g carbohydrate, 8 g fat, 41 mg cholesterol, 8 g dietary fiber, 683 mg sodium.

BEEF STROGANOFF

12 ounces boneless beef sirloin steak, cut ½ to ¾ inch thick
6 ounces packaged dried fettuccine
1 8-ounce carton light dairy sour cream
2 tablespoons all-purpose flour
1 tablespoon low-sodium tomato paste
1 teaspoon instant beef bouillon granules
  Nonstick spray coating
2 cups sliced fresh mushrooms
1 medium onion, chopped (½ cup)
1 clove garlic, minced
1 tablespoon snipped fresh parsley

◆ **Trim** separable fat from beef. Partially freeze beef; thinly slice across the grain into bite-size strips. Cook the fettuccine according to package directions, *except* omit cooking oil and salt; drain well.

◆ **Meanwhile,** combine sour cream, flour, and tomato paste in a small bowl. Stir in bouillon, ½ cup *cold water,* and ⅛ teaspoon *pepper.* Set aside.

◆ **Spray** an unheated large skillet with nonstick coating. Preheat the skillet over medium heat. Add beef; cook and stir 2 to 3 minutes or until beef is desired doneness. Remove beef from the skillet. Add mushrooms, onion, and garlic. Cook and stir 3 to 4 minutes or until onion is tender.

◆ **Add** the sour cream mixture to the skillet. Cook and stir over medium heat until thickened and bubbly. Return meat to the skillet. Cook and stir for 2 minutes more. Serve meat mixture over fettuccine. Sprinkle with parsley. Makes 4 servings.

NUTRITION FACTS PER SERVING: 390 calories, 28 g protein, 49 g carbohydrate, 9 g fat, 57 mg cholesterol, 1 g dietary fiber, 330 mg sodium.

SO LONG, SOUR CREAM

To cut fat and calories in recipes, use an alternative to regular sour cream. Compare 1 ounce (2 tablespoons) of regular sour cream, with its 61 calories and 6 grams fat, to:

• Light dairy sour cream: 37 calories and 2 grams fat
• Fat-free dairy sour cream: 30 calories and 0 grams fat
• Plain low-fat yogurt: 18 calories and .5 grams fat
• Plain fat-free yogurt: 16 calories and 0 grams fat

Note that yogurt may add more of a tangy flavor when substituted for sour cream.

PORK SALAD WITH CABBAGE SLAW

In this delightful warm salad, tender slices of pork are served on top of a mixture of chopped apple and preshredded coleslaw mix, then drizzled with a hot honey-mustard dressing.

        2   boneless pork loin chops, cut 1¼ inches thick
       ¼   teaspoon cracked black pepper
       ⅛   teaspoon ground nutmeg
        5   cups purchased shredded cabbage with carrot (coleslaw mix)
        1   large apple, coarsely chopped
        2   slices turkey bacon *or* bacon
       ⅓   cup cider vinegar
       ⅓   cup apple juice *or* apple cider
        1   tablespoon honey
        2   teaspoons honey-mustard
        1   teaspoon caraway seed
            Apple slices (optional)

◆ **Set** oven to broil. Sprinkle chops with pepper and nutmeg. Place on the unheated rack of a broiler pan. Broil 4 to 5 inches from the heat for 18 to 25 minutes or until no longer pink, turning the chops once.

◆ **Meanwhile,** combine cabbage with carrot and the chopped apple in a large bowl; set aside. Cook bacon in a medium skillet until crisp. Drain bacon, crumble, and set aside.

◆ **Add** vinegar, apple juice, honey, mustard, and caraway seed to skillet. Bring to boiling. Pour over coleslaw mixture; add bacon. Toss to mix.

◆ **Arrange** coleslaw mixture on individual serving plates. Cut pork into ¼-inch-thick slices. Arrange pork slices on top of coleslaw mixture. Garnish with apple slices, if desired. Makes 4 servings.

NUTRITION FACTS PER SERVING: 167 calories, 11 g protein, 20 g carbohydrate, 6 g fat, 30 mg cholesterol, 3 g dietary fiber, 212 mg sodium.

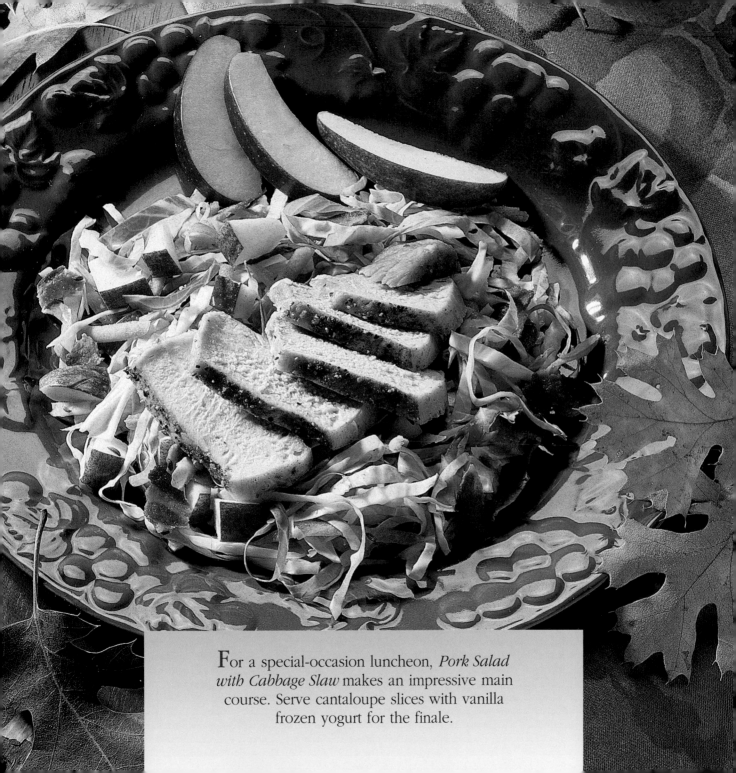

For a special-occasion luncheon, *Pork Salad with Cabbage Slaw* makes an impressive main course. Serve cantaloupe slices with vanilla frozen yogurt for the finale.

PORK WITH PEAR-PEPPERCORN SAUCE

The sweetness of pear nectar balances the sharp flavor of the peppercorns in this elegant entrée. Serve with hot cooked pasta or rice.

2   medium pears, cored and sliced
    Pear nectar *or* orange juice (about 1 cup)
1   tablespoon cooking oil
4   boneless pork loin chops, cut 1 inch thick (12 ounces total)
1   tablespoon all-purpose flour
1   tablespoon Dijon-style mustard
1   teaspoon whole black *or* multi-colored peppercorns, crushed
¼   teaspoon ground nutmeg

◆ **Place** the pear slices in a medium saucepan. Cover with the pear nectar. Bring to boiling; reduce the heat. Simmer, covered, for 5 to 7 minutes or until tender. Remove the pear slices with a slotted spoon, reserving liquid. Cover the pears; keep warm. Measure the liquid; if necessary, add pear nectar to equal *1 cup.* Set aside.

◆ **Meanwhile,** heat the cooking oil in a large skillet over medium-high heat. Add the chops; reduce heat to medium. Cook for 10 to 12 minutes or until the center is just slightly pink, turning once. Remove the chops from skillet, reserving drippings in skillet.

◆ **For sauce,** stir the flour into the drippings. Stir in the reserved pear nectar mixture, the mustard, peppercorns, and nutmeg. Cook and stir until thickened and bubbly. Cook and stir for 1 minute more.

◆ **Place** chops on 4 individual serving plates; arrange pears around chops. Top with sauce; sprinkle with additional pepper. Makes 4 servings.

NUTRITION FACTS PER SERVING: 252 calories, 21 g protein, 26 g carbohydrate, 9 g fat, 50 mg cholesterol, 3 g dietary fiber, 163 mg sodium.

GREEK LAMB STIR-FRY

To save time, purchase prewashed spinach to prepare this vegetable-and-lamb stir-fry.

  8 ounces lean boneless lamb *or* boneless beef top round steak
  3 tablespoons cooking oil
  1 tablespoon lemon juice *or* balsamic vinegar
  ½ teaspoon dried rosemary, crushed
  ½ teaspoon dried oregano, crushed
  ¼ teaspoon pepper
  1 medium carrot, thinly bias sliced (½ cup)
  1 small red onion, thinly sliced
  1 clove garlic, minced
  4 cups purchased torn fresh spinach (about 5 ounces)
  2 small tomatoes, cut into thin wedges
  ¼ cup crumbled feta cheese (1 ounce)

◆ **Trim** fat from lamb; partially freeze. Thinly slice across grain into bite-size strips.

◆ **For sauce,** combine *1 tablespoon* of the oil, the lemon juice, rosemary, oregano, and pepper in a small bowl.

◆ **Pour** *1 tablespoon* oil into a wok or large skillet. Preheat over medium-high heat. Add sliced carrot and onion; stir-fry for 3 to 4 minutes or until crisp-tender. Remove vegetables from wok or skillet.

◆ **Add** remaining oil to wok or skillet. Add lamb and garlic; stir-fry for 2 to 3 minutes or until lamb is brown.

◆ **Return** cooked vegetables to wok or skillet. Add sauce, spinach, and tomatoes. Stir to coat all ingredients with sauce. Remove from heat. Top with cheese. Makes 3 servings.

NUTRITION FACTS PER SERVING: 298 calories, 20 g protein, 11 g carbohydrate, 20 g fat, 57 mg cholesterol, 3 g dietary fiber, 206 mg sodium.

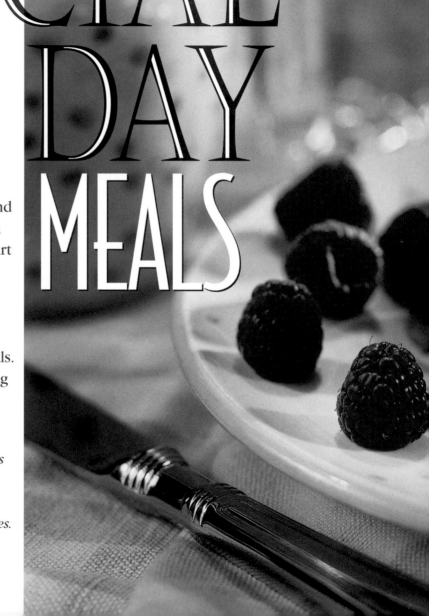

SPECIAL-DAY MEALS

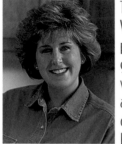

Test kitchen pro Lori Wilson says, "It's easy to pamper your family with great meals on the weekends. All it takes is a little planning, and you can be in and out of the kitchen fast!"

Because spending time around the dinner table (and not in the kitchen!) is an important part of her family life on weekends, *Better Homes and Gardens®* Test Kitchen home economist Lori Wilson created two quick and healthful together-time meals. Shared here are her menus, along with tips for pulling them off with ease.

Weekend mornings are perfect times for Lori to pamper her family with this slow-down-and-savor brunch that she makes special without adding unnecessary fat and calories.

84

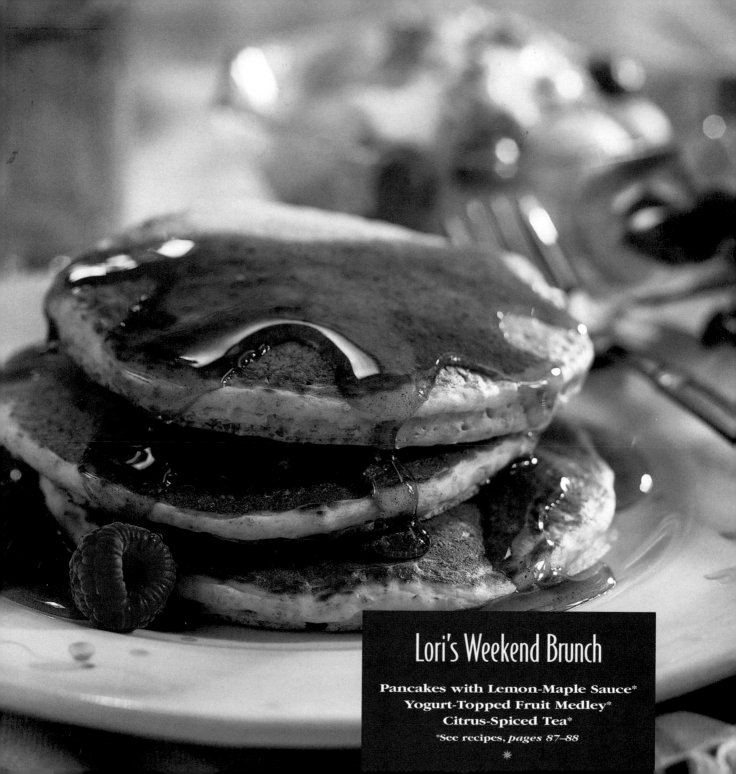

Lori's Weekend Brunch

Pancakes with Lemon-Maple Sauce*
Yogurt-Topped Fruit Medley*
Citrus-Spiced Tea*
*See recipes, *pages 87–88*

SPECIAL-DAY MEALS
TODAY'S COOKING MADE EASY

Countdown

The night before brunch: Place frozen fruit in the refrigerator to thaw.

30 minutes before brunch: Preheat the oven to 200°. Prepare Yogurt-Topped Fruit Medley; chill.

25 minutes before brunch: Prepare pancake batter as directed *opposite*.

20 minutes before brunch: Cook pancakes, then transfer to an ovenproof serving platter. Cover and keep warm in a preheated oven. Meanwhile, prepare the Lemon-Maple Sauce. Keep sauce warm in a saucepan.

5 minutes before brunch: Prepare the Citrus-Spiced Tea.

To serve: Transfer pancake sauce to a small pitcher.

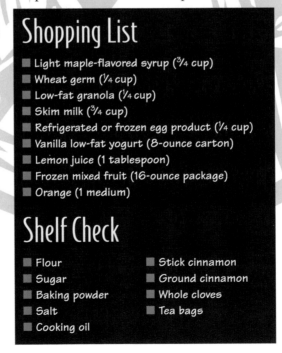

Shopping List

- Light maple-flavored syrup (¾ cup)
- Wheat germ (¼ cup)
- Low-fat granola (¼ cup)
- Skim milk (¾ cup)
- Refrigerated or frozen egg product (¼ cup)
- Vanilla low-fat yogurt (8-ounce carton)
- Lemon juice (1 tablespoon)
- Frozen mixed fruit (16-ounce package)
- Orange (1 medium)

Shelf Check

- Flour
- Sugar
- Baking powder
- Salt
- Cooking oil
- Stick cinnamon
- Ground cinnamon
- Whole cloves
- Tea bags

PANCAKES WITH LEMON-MAPLE SAUCE

One whole egg can be substituted for the refrigerated or frozen egg product; however, the calorie, fat, and cholesterol content of the recipe will increase.

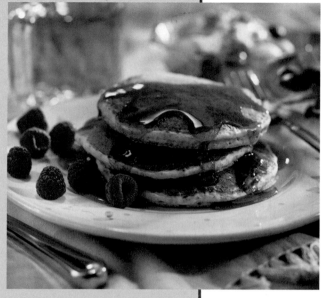

- 1 cup all-purpose flour
- ¼ cup toasted wheat germ
- 1 tablespoon sugar
- 1½ teaspoons baking powder
- ⅛ teaspoon salt
- ¾ cup skim milk
- ¼ cup refrigerated *or* frozen*
      egg product
- 2 teaspoons cooking oil
- ¾ cup light maple-flavored syrup
- 1 tablespoon lemon juice
- ¼ teaspoon ground cinnamon
      Fresh raspberries (optional)

◆ **Combine** flour, wheat germ, sugar, baking powder, and salt in a medium mixing bowl. Combine skim milk, egg product, and oil in a small mixing bowl. Add all at once to flour mixture. Stir just until mixed but still slightly lumpy.

◆ **For** each pancake, pour about *¼ cup* batter onto a hot, lightly greased griddle or heavy skillet. Cook until pancakes are golden brown, turning to cook second side when pancakes have bubbly surfaces and slightly dry edges.

◆ **Meanwhile**, combine syrup, lemon juice, and cinnamon in a small saucepan. Cook over medium heat until heated through, stirring once or twice. Pass syrup mixture with pancakes. Serve with raspberries, if desired. Makes 4 servings.

◆ ***Note:** Thaw egg product, if frozen.

NUTRITION FACTS PER SERVING: 285 calories, 9 g protein, 54 g carbohydrate, 4 g fat, 1 mg cholesterol, 1g dietary fiber, 394 mg sodium.

YOGURT-TOPPED FRUIT MEDLEY

Thaw frozen fruit overnight in the refrigerator or use microwave thawing instructions found on the package.

1 16-ounce package frozen mixed fruit, thawed
1 8-ounce carton vanilla low-fat yogurt
¼ cup low-fat granola

◆ **Spoon** fruit into 4 dessert dishes. Top with yogurt and sprinkle with granola. Makes 4 servings.

NUTRITION FACTS PER SERVING: 184 calories, 4 g protein, 41 g carbohydrate, 2 g fat, 3 mg cholesterol, 2 g dietary fiber, 43 mg sodium.

CITRUS-SPICED TEA

2 inches stick cinnamon
2 2x1-inch strips orange peel with white removed
1 teaspoon whole cloves
3 cups water
2 tea bags

◆ **Place** cinnamon, peel, and cloves on a piece of clean 100% cotton cheesecloth for cooking; tie into a bag. Combine water and the spice bag in a medium saucepan. Bring to boiling; reduce heat. Simmer, covered, for 10 minutes. Remove spice bag and discard.

◆ **Pour** the spiced water mixture over the tea bags in a teapot. Cover the pot and let steep for 5 minutes. Remove the tea bags. Serve at once. Makes 4 (6-ounce) servings.

NUTRITION FACTS PER SERVING: 2 calories, 0 g protein, 1 g carbohydrate, 0 g fat, 0 mg cholesterol, 0 g dietary fiber, 5 mg sodium.

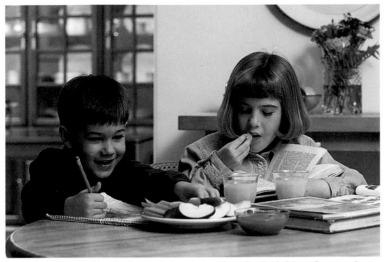

Lori strives to offer healthful foods as snacks. Here, Lori's children, Drew and Jessica, enjoy apple wedges and fat-free caramel sauce.

Smart (and Easy) Snacking

Like the English with their tea-time, and the French with *"le quatre-heures"* (a four-o'clock snack time), Lori offers treats to her family to stave off the between-meal hunger-pangs that occur after school and before dinner. Here are a few of her suggestions for quick and healthful snacks:

◆ Rather than a sugar-filled (and vitamin empty) soda-pop, serve a cool orange sipper: Combine equal parts of orange juice and carbonated water in a glass and add ice cubes.

◆ Keep homemade or purchased bran muffins handy in the freezer. Thaw and serve with mugs of hot low-fat chocolate milk.

◆ For a quick nibble anytime, serve assorted dried fruits.

◆ Satisfy little sweet tooths with unsweetened applesauce sprinkled with raisins. Or, serve apple wedges and fat-free caramel sauce—a favorite at Lori's house.

◆ When the gang comes over for after-school playtime, serve fun finger-foods, such as dill pickle spears wrapped with a slice of lean turkey breast, or flour tortillas sprinkled with low-fat cheese, micro-cooked, then served with salsa for dipping. Cut-up fresh vegetables served with reduced-calorie dressing also make fun and healthful dippers.

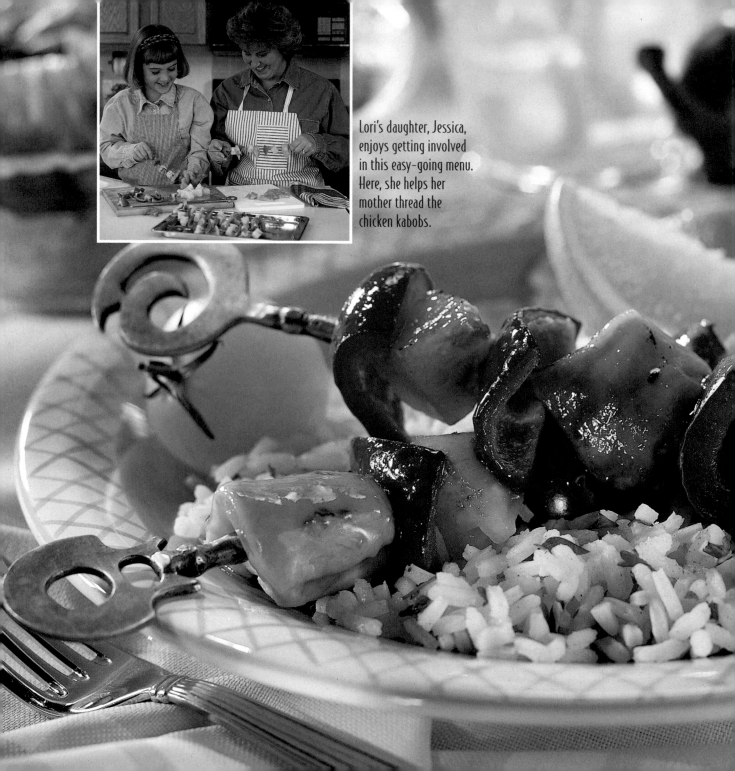

Lori's daughter, Jessica, enjoys getting involved in this easy-going menu. Here, she helps her mother thread the chicken kabobs.

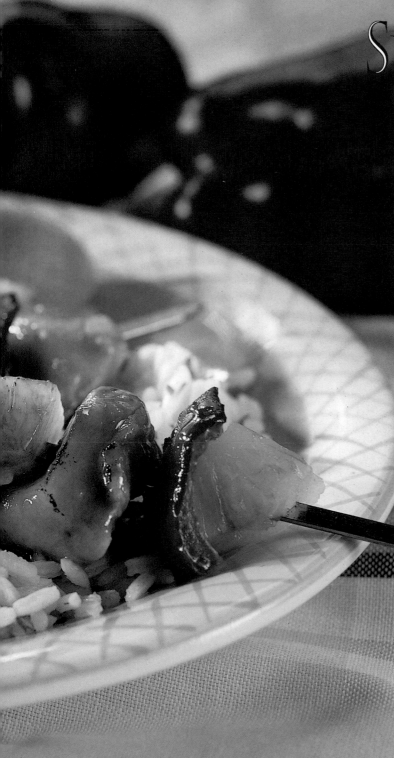

As the work week winds down, Lori gears up for mealtime enjoyment with her family. As in many households, the Wilsons often wait for the weekend to celebrate birthdays, soccer victories, academic achievements, and other special events. She finds that this first-rate menu is right on target with her aim to serve healthful meals to her family, without sacrificing style and pleasure. It also fits perfectly into her schedule, taking only 30 minutes from start to finish.

Lori's Weekend Dinner

Chicken Kabobs with Orange Rice*

Mixed greens salad with fat-free dressing

Caramel Apple Sundaes*

Sparkling water with lemon

*See recipes, *page 93*

＊

SPECIAL-DAY
MEALS
TODAY'S COOKING MADE EASY.

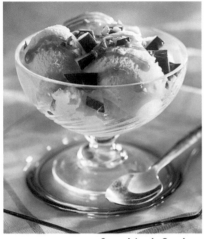

Carmel Apple Sundaes

Countdown

30 minutes before dinner: Transfer salad greens to a salad bowl; chill. Scoop frozen yogurt for Caramel Apple Sundaes into dessert dishes; freeze.

25 minutes before dinner: Preheat broiler. Rinse chicken for Chicken Kabobs and pat dry. Cut up chicken and thread on skewers along with pineapple and pepper.

15 minutes before dinner: Broil kabobs. Prepare basting sauce. Prepare rice mixture.

5 minutes before dinner: Toss salad greens with dressing.

To serve: Transfer rice mixture and kabobs to a serving platter.

Before dessert: Chop apple; assemble Caramel Apple Sundaes. Relax and enjoy!

Shopping List

- Skinless, boneless chicken breast halves (12 ounces)
- Red or green sweet pepper (1 large)
- Fresh parsley (1 bunch)
- Packaged salad greens, prewashed (4 cups)
- Apple (1 small)
- Pineapple chunks, juice pack (8-ounce can)
- Apricot or peach preserves (⅓ cup)
- Vanilla frozen yogurt
- Caramel ice-cream topping

Shelf Check

- Light soy sauce
- Quick-cooking rice
- Fat-free salad dressing
- Orange juice
- Ground ginger
- Ground nutmeg
- Chopped nuts

Chicken Kabobs with Orange Rice

If you assemble the kabobs ahead of time, your meal will come together even quicker. Pictured on pages 90–91.

- 12 ounces skinless, boneless chicken breast halves
- 1 8-ounce can pineapple chunks (juice pack), drained
- 1 large red *or* green sweet pepper, cut into 1-inch pieces
- ⅓ cup apricot preserves *or* peach preserves
- 2 teaspoons light soy sauce
- ⅛ teaspoon ground ginger
- 1½ cups orange juice
- ¼ teaspoon ground nutmeg
- 1½ cups quick-cooking rice
- 1 tablespoon snipped fresh parsley
  Orange wedges (optional)
  Yellow cherry tomatoes (optional)

◆ **Set oven** to broil. Rinse chicken; pat dry with paper towels. Cut chicken into 1-inch pieces. Alternately thread the chicken pieces, pineapple chunks, and pepper pieces on 8 long metal skewers. Place the skewers on the unheated rack of a broiler pan. Broil 4 inches from the heat for 6 minutes.

◆ **Meanwhile**, combine preserves, soy sauce, and ginger in a small bowl. Set aside. Combine orange juice and nutmeg in a medium saucepan. Bring to boiling. Stir in rice. Cover and remove from the heat. Let stand for 5 minutes. Stir in parsley.

◆ **Turn kabobs** and brush with preserve mixture. Broil for 4 minutes more or until chicken is tender and no longer pink and vegetables are of desired doneness. Serve kabobs with rice. Garnish with orange wedges and cherry tomatoes, if desired. Makes 4 servings.

NUTRITION FACTS PER SERVING: 387 calories, 20 g protein, 70 g carbohydrate, 3 g fat, 45 mg cholesterol, 2 g dietary fiber, 137 mg sodium.

Caramel Apple Sundaes

Be sure to measure the caramel sauce—use about 2 teaspoons for each serving. Pictured opposite.

- 1⅓ cups vanilla frozen yogurt
- 3 tablespoons caramel ice-cream topping
- 1 tablespoon chopped nuts
- 1 small apple, cored and chopped

◆ Place about ⅓ *cup* of vanilla frozen yogurt into each of 4 dessert dishes. Top each with some of ice-cream topping and nuts; add chopped apple. Makes 4 servings.

NUTRITION FACTS PER SERVING: 172 calories, 3 g protein, 31 g carbohydrate, 5 g fat, 6 mg cholesterol, 1 g dietary fiber, 92 mg sodium.

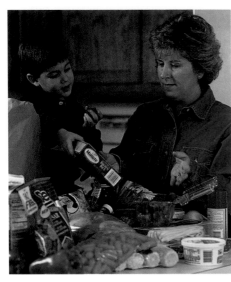

Healthful, fast, and delicious—
to bring these qualities to her
family's table, Lori knows that
smart shopping is a key element
of her plan.

Smart Shopping

Busy cooks know that getting the groceries
sometimes takes more time than cooking meals.
And home economists know that buying the
right ingredients is key to healthful eating.
That's why Lori devised this master plan for
grocery shopping. Here are her major strategies:

◆ Plan menus for several days at a time. This will allow you to shop for
groceries only twice each week.

◆ Leave the children at home. You'll save time and money, and buy fewer junk
foods, if you shop alone.

◆ Don't go to the store when you're hungry. It's much more challenging to
say no to impulse items on an empty stomach.

◆ Make a list, and stick to it, except for seasonal produce and items offered at
special sale prices.

◆ Avoid backtracking by writing your shopping list in the same order that
you walk through the store.

◆ To save time, shop when the store is least likely to be crowded. Lori goes to
the grocery store on weeknights while her husband puts the children to bed
or very early on Saturday mornings.

◆ Read labels and learn as much as you can about the nutritional content of
the foods you buy. Look for as many low-calorie, low-fat, or low-sodium foods
as possible so you can moderate your intake of these nutrients more easily.

A–C

Baked Sole and Corn Salsa 67
Balsamic Chicken with Zucchini 10
BEEF
    Beef Stroganoff 79
    Blackened Beef Stir-Fry 56
    Chili-Mac Skillet 78
    Chunky Potato Chowder 23
    Garden Beef Salad 24
    Greek Lamb Stir-Fry 83
    Pepper Steak 58
    Quick Greek-Style Burritos 22
    Roast Beef and Peppercorn Pitas 24
    Sloppy Joes 59
    Thai Beef Salad 76
Black Beans and Rice 75
Blackened Beef Stir-Fry 56
Broccoli and Pasta, Curried 74
BRUNCH
    Citrus-Spiced Tea 88
    Ham and Asparagus Omelets 25
    Pancakes with Lemon-Maple Sauce . .87
    Yogurt-Topped Fruit Medley 88
Bulgur Skillet, Chicken 36
Burritos, Quick Greek-Style 22
Caramel Apple Sundaes 93
Cheese Ravioli with Zucchini Sauce 20
CHICKEN
    Balsamic Chicken with Zucchini 10
    Chicken à la King 29
    Chicken and Feta Salad-
        Stuffed Pitas 12
    Chicken and Fettuccine with
        Mustard Sauce 12
    Chicken and Orange Stir-Fry 44
    Chicken and Raspberry
        Spinach Salad 66
    Chicken and Tropical Fruit Plate 39

CHICKEN (cont'd.)

    Chicken Bulgur Skillet 36
    Chicken Cacciatore 62
    Chicken Kabobs with Orange Rice . . .93
    Chicken Parmigiana 28
    Chicken with Cherry Sauce 30
    Chicken with Salsa Couscous 34
    Chunky Potato Chowder 23
    Glazed Chicken and Grapes 8
    Herbed Chicken Sandwiches 6
    Hoisin Broiled Chicken
        with Cashews 8
    Italian Turkey Burgers 38
    Lemon-Pepper Chicken with
        Mushroom Sauce 37
    Linguine with Chicken and
        Clam Sauce 33
    Mango Chicken 64
    Quick Chicken Oriental 32
    Roasted Italian Chicken and
        Vegetables 63
    Saffron Chicken and Rice 11
    Tex-Mex Chicken Tostadas 6
    Turkey with Tropical Fruit Salsa 14
    Waldorf Turkey Salad with
        Cantaloupe 42
    Zesty Fried Chicken 7
Chili-Mac Skillet 78
Chili-Sauced Pasta 20
Chili with Biscuits, Vegetarian 72
Chowder, Chunky Potato 23
Chowder, Manhattan Clam 51
Chunky Potato Chowder 23
Citrus-Spiced Tea 88
Clam Chowder, Manhattan 51
Clam Sauce, Linguine with
    Chicken and 33
Crab Salad, Curried 16

Crunchy Oven-Fried Fish 16
Curried Broccoli and Pasta 74
Curried Crab Salad 16

D–K

DESSERTS
    Caramel Apple Sundaes 93
FISH AND SEAFOOD
    Baked Sole and Corn Salsa 67
    Crunchy Oven-Fried Fish 16
    Curried Crab Salad 16
    Flounder Dijon 68
    Fruit and Tuna Salad 18
    Halibut with Garden-Style
        Marinara Sauce 46
    Lemony Fish Fillets 18
    Linguine with Chicken and
        Clam Sauce 33
    Manhattan Clam Chowder 51
    Pasta Primavera with Salmon 43
    Roasted Red Snapper 70
    Sole with Spinach and Plum
        Tomatoes 47
    Sunshine Shrimp 50
    Tarragon Shrimp 19
    Turkey and Shrimp Jambalaya 48
Flounder Dijon 68
Fruit and Tuna Salad 18
Fruit Salsa, Turkey with Tropical 14
Garden Beef Salad 24
Glazed Chicken and Grapes 8
Greek Lamb Stir-Fry 83
Halibut with Garden-Style
    Marinara Sauce 46
Ham and Asparagus Omelets 25
Herbed Chicken Sandwiches 6
Hoisin Broiled Chicken with Cashews 8
Italian Turkey Burgers 38

L–R

LAMB
Greek Lamb Stir-Fry 83
Mint-Glazed Lamb Chops 22
Lemon-Pepper Chicken with
Mushroom Sauce 37
Lemony Fish Fillets 18
Linguine with Chicken and
Clam Sauce 33
Mango Chicken 64
Manhattan Clam Chowder 51

MEATLESS DISHES
Black Beans and Rice 75
Cheese Ravioli with
Zucchini Sauce 20
Chili-Sauced Pasta 20
Curried Broccoli and Pasta 74
Vegetarian Chili with Biscuits 72
Mint-Glazed Lamb Chops 22
Omelets, Ham and Asparagus 25
Pancakes with Lemon-Maple Sauce 87

PASTA
Cheese Ravioli with
Zucchini Sauce 20
Chicken and Fettuccine with
Mustard Sauce 12
Chicken Cacciatore 62
Chili-Mac Skillet 78
Chili-Sauced Pasta 20
Curried Broccoli and Pasta 74
Linguine with Chicken and
Clam Sauce 33
Pasta Primavera with Salmon 43
Pepper Steak 58
Picatta-Style Pork 54
Pitas, Chicken and Feta Salad-Stuffed . .12
Pitas, Roast Beef and Peppercorn 24

PORK
Ham and Asparagus Omelets 25
Picatta-Style Pork 54

PORK (cont'd.)
Pork Medaillons with Apple-Yogurt
Sauce .52
Pork Salad with Cabbage Slaw 80
Pork with Pear-Peppercorn Sauce . . .82
Wine-Sauced Pork Medaillons 55
Quick Chicken Oriental 32
Quick Greek-Style Burritos 22
Ravioli with Zucchini Sauce, Cheese . . .20
Red Snapper, Roasted 70
Rice, Black Beans and 75
Roast Beef and Peppercorn Pitas 24
Roasted Italian Chicken and Vegetables . . .63
Roasted Red Snapper 70

S–Z

Saffron Chicken and Rice 11

SALADS
Chicken and Raspberry
Spinach Salad 66
Chicken and Tropical Fruit Plate 39
Curried Crab Salad 16
Fruit and Tuna Salad 18
Garden Beef Salad 24
Pork Salad with Cabbage Slaw 80
Thai Beef Salad 76
Waldorf Turkey Salad with
Cantaloupe 42
Salmon, Pasta Primavera with 43
Salsa, Baked Sole and Corn 67

SANDWICHES
Chicken and Feta Salad-
Stuffed Pitas 12
Herbed Chicken Sandwiches 6
Italian Turkey Burgers 38
Quick Greek-Style Burritos 22
Roast Beef and Peppercorn Pitas 24
Sloppy Joes 59
Tex-Mex Chicken Tostadas 6
Sautéed Turkey with Tomatoes 15
Shrimp Jambalaya, Turkey and 48

Shrimp, Sunshine 50
Shrimp, Tarragon 19
Sloppy Joes 59
Sole and Corn Salsa, Baked 67
Sole with Spinach and
Plum Tomatoes 47
Spinach Salad, Chicken and
Raspberry 66
Sunshine Shrimp 50
Tarragon Shrimp 19
Tea, Citrus-Spiced 88
Tex-Mex Chicken Tostadas 6
Thai Beef Salad 76
Tostadas, Tex-Mex Chicken 6
Tuna Salad, Fruit and 18

TURKEY
Chicken à la King 29
Chunky Potato Chowder 23
Hoisin Broiled Chicken with
Cashews 8
Italian Turkey Burgers 38
Linguine with Chicken and
Clam Sauce 33
Quick Chicken Oriental 32
Sautéed Turkey with Tomatoes 15
Turkey and Shrimp Jambalaya 48
Turkey Apricot Stir-Fry 69
Turkey Marsala 40
Turkey Sauté with Mustard Sauce 14
Turkey with Tropical Fruit Salsa 14
Waldorf Turkey Salad with
Cantaloupe 42
Vegetarian Chili with Biscuits 72
Waldorf Turkey Salad with Cantaloupe 42
Wine-Sauced Pork Medaillons 55
Yogurt-Topped Fruit Medley 88
Zesty Fried Chicken 7